Chicken Soup for the Dieter's Soul®

Daily Inspirations

Jack Canfield
Mark Victor Hansen
Patricia Lorenz

Health Communica
Deerfield Beach,

www.hcibooks
www.chickenso

D0169838

The following recipes were originally published in *Chicken Soup for the Soul Cookbook, 101 Recipes from the Heart*. ©1995 Jack Canfield, Mark Victor Hansen, Diana von Welanetz Wentworth.

Neighborhood Soup (March 8). Reprinted by permission of Linda McNamar. ©1995 Linda McNamar.

Health Nut Pancakes (October 11). Reprinted by permission of Rama J. Vernon. ©1995 Rama J. Vernon.

Fresh Horseradish (November 21). Reprinted by permission of Theodore Wentworth. ©1995 Theodore Wentworth.

**Library of Congress Cataloging-in-Publication Data
is available from the Library of Congress.**

©2006 Jack Canfield and Mark Victor Hansen
ISBN-13: 978-0-7573-0526-9
ISBN-10: 0-7573-0526-1

Publisher: Health Communications, Inc.
            3201 S.W. 15th Street
            Deerfield Beach, FL 33442-8190

Cover and inside design by Larissa Hise Henoch
Inside book formatting by Theresa Peluso

We dedicate this book to
everyone striving for
better health;
mentally, physically
and spiritually.

Introduction

This is not a diet book. This is a book about inspiration, motivation and celebration. It's a book with big ideas and big goals. It's a book about better health, a happier life, more energy and hope for the future. It's a book about changing habits and patterns that will be lifelong.

Overeating and underexercising has a powerful hold on many of us. I have been trying to lose weight most of my life, and I think many people struggle with weight issues. Being at a healthy weight is an important part of taking care of ourselves. Just as important is becoming the best person we can be, and learning to love ourselves, forgive ourselves and energize ourselves.

When my daughter Julia was in college majoring in health promotion and wellness, she knew I was trying (again) to lose weight and exercise more. Always supportive of my attempts to improve my health and fitness, Julia shared a concept she thought would help me reach my objective. "Each letter in the word **SPECIES** represents a different area of a truly healthy being. *Social, Physical, Emotional, Career, Intellectual, Environmental* and *Spiritual.* We have to make all the parts work in order to be truly healthy, Mom."

I've kept those seven keys close to my heart ever since. You'll read about them throughout this book as we work together to create a life that brims with good health.

Thank you for taking this journey with me. Getting healthy by *eating better, eating less* and *exercising more* could possibly be the toughest thing we ever do. But if we keep at it every day, we'll discover that being healthy, happy and hopeful is our reward for making some simple lifestyle changes.

Open your heart and pour out your feelings on the lines provided on each page. Journaling is an amazing way to know that our minds and bodies are changing for the better.

And remember, it's one day at a time. Baby steps. New ideas. New habits. New lifestyle. We're in this together. And we can do this. We can get healthy. We can be fit, have fun, be happy, hopeful and full of energy. I believe this with all my heart. Let's begin!

Patricia Lorenz

For most of my adult life I've made *lose weight* my New Year's resolution. This year is different. This year, it's get healthy by making a commitment to eat better foods, less of them and to exercise more. It seems like a lifelong plan and not a diet. Let's do it together. The way I look at it, these bodies of ours are a gift and it's our responsibility to cherish them and keep them healthy.

Tonight when we undress, let's turn around slowly in front of the mirror. Look at that belly fat and/or those roly-poly hips and thighs.

Let's promise ourselves to get healthy by *eating better, eating less* and *exercising more.* Ladies and gentlemen, start your engines!

DIETER'S DELIGHTS & DILEMMAS

JANUARY 2

If you're like me you hate to throw away perfectly good food, but sometimes that's the best thing we can do for our health.

This time of year I look at all the holiday cookies, cakes and candies. It's hard to just toss it all out. But then when I look at my goals for this year, I know that getting rid of all those white flour calories and fat is the best thing I can do for my body.

So out they go! Hopefully this year we'll be able to find many ways to make sure that all the food we put in our mouths is not only delicious but very nutritious as well.

DIETER'S DELIGHTS & DILEMMAS

_____

_____

_____

_____

_____

_____

_____

_____

_____

_____

We may be asking ourselves, *What exactly does eating better mean?* Simple, just take all those articles we've read and the hundreds of TV shows we've watched about nutrition and fitness, and put that knowledge to work. We both know what *eat better* means. It means 100 percent whole-grain breads and pastas. Brown rice. Non- or low-fat milk, yogurt, cheese and salad dressings. It means eliminating most white sugar, white flour and high-fat products. Eating more fresh fruits and brightly colored vegetables. Less red meat. Healthy snacks.

We know the drill. We know what it means. We know which aisles to avoid in the grocery store. We already know and **now we're really going to do it.**

DIETER'S DELIGHTS & DILEMMAS

_____

_____

_____

_____

_____

_____

_____

_____

_____

_____

Remember the word **SPECIES** from the introduction. It's an acronym that represents the seven essential elements to a truly healthy being:

Social

Physical

Emotional

Career

Intellectual

Environmental

Spiritual

As we work hard this year on the physical part of wellness, let's also study up on the other six. Just think what an amazingly wonderful **SPECIES** we'll be by December 31!

DIETER'S DELIGHTS & DILEMMAS

For thirty-two years, my dad, who was born in 1919, was a rural mail carrier. Every year for Christmas his patrons gave him, in addition to about twenty bottles of aftershave, boxes and bags full of candy and cookies. The chocolate-covered cherries were my favorites. And every year in January, Dad started writing thank-you letters for each and every gift.

Today, let's write someone a handwritten thank-you letter. "Thank you, Mary, for being my walking partner and for helping me gets in shape."

"Thank you, Alice, for reminding me to eat more salads and fewer desserts. I treasure your help with my new fitness plan."

Get out the pen and paper and make someone's day.

DIETER'S DELIGHTS & DILEMMAS

_____

_____

_____

_____

_____

_____

_____

_____

_____

_____

JANUARY 6

I learned years ago that clutter is not my friend. When my home is neat and things are relatively organized, I feel so much better.

I've also learned that to stay on a healthy-eating plan and get into the habit of daily exercise, my surroundings have to be healthy as well. So today, let's put away all the holiday decorations. But let's only put out half of the usual knickknacks.

I've learned that a simpler life helps me stay on track when it comes to making new habits. One of those is walking. It's easy, free and perfect for those of us who are just starting to exercise again. Take a brisk walk today. Do it again tomorrow. See how many miles you can walk by the end of the month.

DIETER'S DELIGHTS & DILEMMAS

Who says we have to give up our favorite treats just because we're trying to lose weight and get healthy?

I love almonds, especially chocolate-covered almonds. And since almonds are among the best nuts we can eat, I buy reduced-salt almonds and a small bag of chocolate-covered almonds every few months. For a mid-afternoon snack once a week or so, I'll eat five of the chocolate ones and ten of the reduced-salt ones.

It's a grand treat combining all three of the things we crave: **sweet, salty, crunchy**. But the secret is keeping the portions to a manageable, healthy size.

DIETER'S DELIGHTS & DILEMMAS

_____

_____

_____

_____

_____

_____

_____

_____

_____

JANUARY 8

It may be cold out, but bundle up and get some exercise outdoors. Nothing relieves midwinter blahs better than being outside in the fresh air and sunshine.

Whether you're sledding, skating or snow-skiing up north . . . or biking, walking or playing golf down south, just getting outside is a great stress reliever. Whether you're shoveling snow or pulling weeds, moving around outdoors is great for your circulation.

Fresh-air exercise lightens your mood as well.

It doesn't matter if it's 75 degrees where you live or 5 below zero; either way, open that door and enjoy the great outdoors.

DIETER'S DELIGHTS & DILEMMAS

_____

_____

_____

_____

_____

_____

_____

_____

_____

_____

What? You noticed your belt is a little loose this morning? Fabulous! Reward yourself with a new bottle of body cream or lotion with a calming scent.

Smooth it on your winter-dry skin. I have some thick face cream my friend Shirley bought for me in Italy that contains olive oil. When I rub it on my forehead and cheeks, I feel younger and radiant. Even if your skin doesn't feel dry, give yourself a creamy rubdown anyway.

Remember, our goal this year is a healthier allover body, and our skin is the biggest organ in our body. Take care of it.

DIETER'S DELIGHTS & DILEMMAS

As I was struggling through my own overweight miseries and feeling grumpy because I hadn't done so well that day, I observed a waitress at a gala banquet I was attending. I watched her attend to everyone's needs with a giant smile. I finally pulled her aside and said, "Debbie, you are one of the happiest people I've ever seen. I just wanted you to know how much I appreciate your work, and I'm also going to mention it to your boss."

Well, Debbie's face lit up like a moonbeam as she stammered one thank you after another. Her delight caused me to feel better than I had all week. Try it. Complimenting another is the best medicine for whatever ails us.

DIETER'S DELIGHTS & DILEMMAS

_____

_____

_____

_____

_____

_____

_____

_____

_____

M y oldest daughter lives in the hills near San Francisco. Jeanne, who has a healthy appetite, has been thin her entire life.

I suspect her high metabolism is due to the energy she expends just getting to and from her house. After parking her car she has to walk up 167 steps to her house or up a steep path that meanders a half-mile from the road.

Today, let's park our car six blocks from our destination and walk the rest of the way. Or ride a bike to work. Take the steps instead of the elevator. Walk to the co-worker's office instead of phoning or e-mailing. Shake, rattle and roll! The ways to get thinner are all around us.

DIETER'S DELIGHTS & DILEMMAS

_____

_____

_____

_____

_____

_____

_____

_____

_____

_____

JANUARY 12

I blew it today. I ate half a bag of bridge mix. What's with these chocolate cravings? Okay, I promise not to beat myself up every time I fall off the wagon.

Tomorrow is just a few hours away. Another chance to take a long, fast walk. Another chance to drink lots of water.

Tomorrow I'm going to buy a dozen things in the produce section, and I'll make the biggest, healthiest salad ever. And I'll invite my friend Brenda over to help me eat it. She's also trying to lose weight. Her son is getting married in September, and she's calling it "the wedding fitness plan."

Marriage is for life, and so is this eating plan!

DIETER'S DELIGHTS & DILEMMAS

_____

_____

_____

_____

_____

_____

_____

_____

_____

_____

O h what a salad! It was so good, I just have to share it with you. I'm going to buy a salad-crisper so I can make a large batch every few days. Then I'll always have a ready-made, healthy meal in an instant. Substitute or add other fresh vegetables you enjoy that are available in your produce department.

For dessert Brenda and I split a small container of fat-free, carmel-flavored yogurt with a bit of nonfat whipped cream.

Now we're cookin'. I'm glad I don't feel the least bit deprived as I change my eating habits. I feel so much better about me and about life, and about my determination to make this new health plan work.

AWESOME SALAD

½ package each fresh spinach, romaine and leaf lettuce
1 each red, green and yellow bell peppers
½ cup each red onion, broccoli, carrots, cauliflower and
     fresh mushrooms
1 (6-ounce) can olives (black or green, or mix them up!)

1. *Wash and dry the vegetables and drain the olives.*
2. *Slice the peppers thinly, lengthwise and chop the other ingredients into bite-size pieces.*
3. *Mix all the ingredients and store in the refrigerator in an airtight container (it will stay fresh for days).*
4. *When you're ready to serve, top with a sprinkling of*
        Grated cheddar cheese, sunflower or sesame seeds,
          or sliced almonds and low-calorie dressing

*Makes about
6 servings*

JANUARY 14

It's never too late to start an exercise program, just like it's never too late to take music lessons. Studies have shown that music lessons dramatically improve reasoning skills needed for math and science.

Music strengthens the links between brain neurons and increases spatial reasoning by 46 percent. Physical exercise provides as dramatic a benefit for our physical bodies as music does for our brains.

As adults, we need to make daily physical exercise our priority. It's a simple fact. Our health improves drastically once we get in the exercise habit . . . and that's music to our ears.

DIETER'S DELIGHTS & DILEMMAS

Today is Dr. Martin Luther King, Jr.'s birthday. One of my all-time favorite quotes came from Dr. King:

"If a man is called to be a streetsweeper, he should sweep streets even as Michelangelo painted, or Beethoven composed music, or Shakespeare wrote poetry. He should sweep streets so well that all the hosts of heaven and earth will pause to say, 'Here lived a great streetsweeper who did his job well.'"

Today I am going to do my job well. I am going to eat healthy foods. I am going to eat smaller portions.

I am going to walk on the treadmill and think about the freedoms that Dr. King helped bring to our country.

DIETER'S DELIGHTS & DILEMMAS

_____

_____

_____

_____

_____

_____

_____

_____

_____

_____

Tonight take a look outside. See any stars up there? A star is nothing more than a self-luminous, self-contained mass of gas.

From earth, a twinkling star can light the way and make all seem right with the world. Now, let's take a look at the stars in our own lives, right here on earth.

It's time to bring them close and let them know that we're trying to *eat better, eat less* and *exercise more.* It's time to tell our families and fitness allies how much we appreciate their support.

Let's ask them to send their success ideas and encouragement our way. We need an army here!

DIETER'S DELIGHTS & DILEMMAS

_____

_____

_____

_____

_____

_____

_____

_____

_____

I s today one of those cold, gray-sky days? I almost put on my old navy flop suit this morning, the one that's paint stained, big enough for two and the most unflattering thing in my closet.

Wearing it makes me want to eat a whole bag of family-size chips and top it off with a bag of malted milk balls. So, I get it. I won't wear the flop suit anymore.

I'll dress nice, pull in my stomach, stand tall and look like a woman on a mission. My mission? To make changes this year that will last a lifetime.

A lifetime of fun, fitness and fabulous health.

DIETER'S DELIGHTS & DILEMMAS

_____

_____

_____

_____

_____

_____

_____

_____

_____

_____

JANUARY 18

I love public speaking because I feel passionate about so many things. One of my favorite topics is *Follow Your Dreams While You're Still Awake*. Some people get so busy raising families and nurturing careers that they forget to nourish their own dreams. One of my life-long dreams was to live in a warm climate near a body of water where I could swim every day. After raising my children and living twenty-four years in Milwaukee, I moved to Florida and bought a small condo.

Because I'm living my dream, I can now concentrate on fine-tuning my life . . . and finally, after trying for so many years, actually get healthier, fitter, thinner. Do you have dreams that need tending?

DIETER'S DELIGHTS & DILEMMAS

_____

_____

_____

_____

_____

_____

_____

_____

_____

_____

When I lived in Wisconsin, January was one of my least favorite months. I'd split wood for the woodburner, pile on layer after layer of clothing, shiver under the covers and eat like a whale working on an extra layer of blubber.

Now that I'm biking and swimming in January in my new warm-climate home, I love hearing from my kids who still live up north, about their winter adventures: sledding, ice skating, and frosty walks in the snow. Whether we live in the frozen tundra or the tropical sunshine, we can take advantage of a thousand ways to exercise. Just get out there. Doesn't matter if we're wearing a parka or a bikini, open the front door and start moving.

DIETER'S DELIGHTS & DILEMMAS

I make lists of everything. Chores to do. Groceries to buy. Foods to avoid. Gifts to give. Places to visit. Lists keep me on track and give me a feeling of accomplishment when I check off the completed items.

Today let's make a list of nine things we can do that will help us meet our goals of *eating better, eating less* and *exercising more.*

Here's the start of my list:

Today I will give away all the white flour products in my pantry.

Today I will eat half of my sandwich at noon and the other half for my 3:30 snack.

Today I will walk a mile with an elderly friend to make *her* feel better, not me.

DIETER'S DELIGHTS & DILEMMAS

_____

_____

_____

_____

_____

_____

_____

_____

_____

_____

D on't you love the word *survivor*? We're all survivors in our own way. I grew up in a happy, two-parent family, but I was married, divorced and annulled twice, and then raised my four children as a single parent for the next seventeen years.

I became a *survivor* because I started to think of myself as the happiest person I knew. It was a matter of attitude adjustment. I was thankful for my children, home, friends, job, woodburner, neighbor who used his snowblower on my driveway, my new roof, chocolate-covered toffee, my old beat-up car that kept chugging, my bicycle and the walking paths along the lake.

Today, let's make a new list of things we're thankful for.

DIETER'S DELIGHTS & DILEMMAS

_____

_____

_____

_____

_____

_____

_____

_____

_____

_____

JANUARY 22

When I was living in Wisconsin, one day the temperature was five below zero and the battery in my car was dead. A gentleman in the parking lot came over and said, "I've got jumper cables." A few minutes later my car was running. When I offered to pay him, he said, "No, thanks. But maybe someday you can help someone else."

A month later I heard this announcement in a store: "There's a customer in the parking lot with a dead battery. If anyone has jumper cables and can help. . . . " I put on my gloves and headed outside to try out my new jumper cables. Paying it forward. What a healthy concept. Remember, we're trying to be healthier mentally as well as physically.

DIETER'S DELIGHTS & DILEMMAS

_____

_____

_____

_____

_____

_____

_____

_____

_____

_____

A s one of the first baby boomers ever born, I've lived long enough to know that good health and a beautiful body are not attained by going on one diet after another. In fact, you won't hear me mention the word *diet* very often in this book. Good health and a beautiful body are the results of a whole package of goods.

To our basic three of **eating better, eating less** and **exercising more,** we can add reducing stress, making friends, expressing gratitude for little things, smiling, standing tall, giving to others and sharing our bounty to the ingredients for good health and a beautiful body. Look in the mirror. Stand tall. Smile. My, aren't we something great?

DIETER'S DELIGHTS & DILEMMAS

_____

_____

_____

_____

_____

_____

_____

_____

_____

_____

My friend Jack, a widower who lives fifty-seven steps from me, is a good man . . . kind, sincere, fun. I've been single since 1985 and have met many guys who ragged about their ex-wives and past lives.

By the time they'd ask for my phone number, I'd give them the Dial-A-Prayer number and be on my way. They taught me that if we moan and groan about our past failures, we can't work on making our future successes happen.

I'm not going to whine about the fact that I haven't exercised for three days. What I will do is ask Jack if he'd like to go for a bike ride this afternoon.

Let's write today's exercise and food goals down here.

DIETER'S DELIGHTS & DILEMMAS

_____

_____

_____

_____

_____

_____

_____

_____

_____

_____

The drive-through burger place near my home makes the best bacon-Swiss-cheeseburger imaginable. I could easily eat one a week. But I don't because I like my arteries just the way they are . . . flowable. But once every three or four months—that's three or four a year—I do enjoy one.

How does that fit into my health plan? I call it the *deny-don't-deny plan.* I deny myself the fries and the full-sugar cola but I enjoy that burger to the max. Three or four times a year won't kill me.

So you see? This plan isn't so hard. It's about being sensible. A burger a week is not sensible.

We want to be good looking AND healthy, right?

DIETER'S DELIGHTS & DILEMMAS

_____

_____

_____

_____

_____

_____

_____

_____

_____

_____

Having once been married to an alcoholic, I'm very sensitive to what alcohol can do to a person. One of the best lines I've ever heard is: "Remember, alcohol gave you wings to fly but then it took away the sky."

Don't you think food binges and overeating do the same thing to those of us who are trying to get healthy by losing weight? Our candy binges, overeating in restaurants, having second helpings and shoving down the salt-and-sugar party foods may give us wings for a few minutes, but then our binges turn our blue skies into guilt, depression, anger and hopelessness. Today, let's stay on track no matter what and keep our skies blue and intact.

DIETER'S DELIGHTS & DILEMMAS

_____

_____

_____

_____

_____

_____

_____

_____

_____

_____

Mozart was born on this day in 1756. Do you think anyone will remember you 250 years after you were born? My grandmother died in the 1930s long before I was born, but her legacy of loving education (she taught college-level math and physics in 1908) will surely last hundreds of years since nearly all of her ancestors are college graduates.

What legacy will we pass down to generations after we're gone? Our dieting prowess? Probably not. But our willingness to become better, stronger, more interesting and more compassionate beings will surely follow us for generations.

Write down the legacies you want to pass on.

DIETER'S DELIGHTS & DILEMMAS

_____

_____

_____

_____

_____

_____

_____

_____

_____

_____

Today is National Kazoo Day. A kazoo is a funny thing. When the strange noises fill a room, laughter follows.

The same thing happens when you share comfort food with friends and family. How about inviting some people over for a potluck dinner? Remind them that you've begun a get-healthy-lose-weight, lifelong adventure and ask them to bring healthy foods to your party.

Enjoy the friendship and warmth of having supportive people in your life.

And remember, laughter is a shortcut to good health.

DIETER'S DELIGHTS & DILEMMAS

_____

_____

_____

_____

_____

_____

_____

_____

_____

_____

My favorite exercises are bike riding and swimming. But the pool across the street is outdoors and there are many weeks when it's too cold to swim, even in my neck of the woods. Same for biking.

So, today, I'm going to open my mind a crack and make a list of other forms of exercise I can get: Line dancing once a week, using the exercise bike or treadmill inside the condo clubhouse and fast-walking outdoors—a great way to meet the neighbors. How about horseback riding, kayaking or in-line skating?

And if you purchased one of those exercise machines advertised on TV, why don't you stop using it for a clothes rack and actually use it for exercising?

DIETER'S DELIGHTS & DILEMMAS

_____

_____

_____

_____

_____

_____

_____

_____

_____

JANUARY 30

I had a few girlfriends over to play board games while their men stayed home to watch the Super Bowl. Unfortunately, the women brought mostly junk food. I'd eaten a salad for dinner, knowing I'd want my share of the belly-fat producers. But I'm happy to say I did not eat one chip.

If you can give up one or two things for most of your life, make it chips and pastries. Both are loaded with fat, the bad kind, and neither has much nutritional value. I admit I eat an apple fritter every six months or so, but that's the whole point of our new health plan. We don't have to feel guilty and give up everything.

We just have to **eat better, eat less, exercise more.**

DIETER'S DELIGHTS & DILEMMAS

_____

_____

_____

_____

_____

_____

_____

_____

_____

_____

L ife is full of choices. Should I take that new job or stay where I am? Should I join that women's group or stay with my old friends?

Should I go back to school or spend more time with my family? Should I marry that guy, look for someone new, or love my single life? Should I eat that candy bar or the nonfat yogurt? Should I watch this TV show or go for a fast walk?

Ask yourself—which choice will make me a better, more interesting, healthier person?

Sometimes that's all it takes and we suddenly find ourselves lacing up our walking shoes and heading out the door.

DIETER'S DELIGHTS & DILEMMAS

_____

_____

_____

_____

_____

_____

_____

_____

_____

_____

MONTHLY CHECK-IN

Goals Achieved _____

_____

_____

_____

Triggers Pulled and Buttons Pushed_____

_____

_____

_____

Effective Strategies_____

_____

_____

_____

TALE OF THE TAPE

	Current	Last	Net Loss/Gain
Weight	_____	_____	_____
Hips	_____	_____	_____
Thighs	_____	_____	_____
Arms	_____	_____	_____
Waist	_____	_____	_____
Bust	_____	_____	_____

The Apostle Paul wrote letters from prison. At the end of one he warned, "Stop being mean, bad-tempered and angry." Haven't we all had days when we feel angry, short-tempered, even downright mean? We take everything out on our kids, spouse, roommate or co-workers. I've learned that those nasty qualities often appear when I'm tired or hungry. I can snap at the person I love the most over the dumbest thing if I haven't eaten for three or four hours. Our bodies, brains and emotions need regular, well-balanced food to function.

As we make it through this year of healthy decisions, let's put good sleep and well-balanced meals at the top of our to-do list. No fair skipping meals!

DIETER'S DELIGHTS & DILEMMAS

February 2

One of my favorite movies is *Groundhog Day*. Bill Murray's character, Phil, is a weatherman who gets trapped in a time loop where he is destined to relive the same experiences until he changes his outlook. While that was good comedic relief, it's not much fun in real life. Changing my outlook changes the outcome!

Whether Phil gets good news today or not, I have great hope for a better, healthier, slimmer body by the end of this year. I can't wait to see the new me!

Anyway, Happy Groundhog Day. Don't let winter get you down. Stay with the program!

DIETER'S DELIGHTS & DILEMMAS

_____

_____

_____

_____

_____

_____

_____

_____

_____

_____

Whe are important people. Perhaps I need to put that in bold print: **We are important.** There is only one person exactly like you in the whole world. We've been given all the gifts we need to become the absolute best people we were intended to be.

We have strength of character. Determination. Intelligence. Willingness to learn. The power to forgive and be forgiven. We have the ability to say no to ice cream, candy bars, grease-bomb hamburgers, shakes, sodas, fries, pies and even malted milk balls. We are smart enough to walk in that grocery store and spend most of our money in the produce section. We are amazing, aren't we?

DIETER'S DELIGHTS & DILEMMAS

_____

_____

_____

_____

_____

_____

_____

_____

_____

Let's talk about drinking. Our plan for life, which includes eating sensibly and moving our bodies in healthy ways, also includes taking in lots and lots of liquids. Most of those liquids should be water. Pure H_2O. It's the best liquid you can pour down your gullet. What's wrong with juice, you ask? Nothing, but instead of eight ounces of orange juice, why not really add to your full feeling and fiber quota and eat two whole oranges instead?

If you're a cola nut and don't like the diet sodas, buy the smaller six-ounce size and only have one 100-calorie can every few days as a special treat. Better yet, drink water and enjoy those 100 calories in a hearty granola bar.

DIETER'S DELIGHTS & DILEMMAS

I remember an instructor asking the class to write down our three favorite things about our own bodies. I looked down at my protruding stomach and my huge calves that look like inverted bowling pins. My face is just average. Hair, a mousy blond. It was the toughest assignment I'd ever had. I thought, *There isn't much I like about my body.* Finally I wrote that my nose was okay; my body, although overweight, was at least reasonably proportionate; and I liked my height, 5'7½".

Today, let's write down five things we like about our bodies. If we keep our positives in mind, it'll be easier to re-do the negatives.

Best foot forward!

DIETER'S DELIGHTS & DILEMMAS

_____

_____

_____

_____

_____

_____

_____

_____

_____

_____

FEBRUARY 6

The Gettysburg Address contains 226 words, the Ten Commandments, 297 words. But the U.S. Department of Agriculture directive on pricing cabbage weighs in at 15,629 words.

Today I'd just like to say a few words. *Thank you.* Thank you for hanging in here with me. It is so hard to stay with a good healthy-eating plan by myself. For most of my entire life, I've eaten too much, too often and sometimes even the wrong kinds of foods. But knowing there are friends out there, people I haven't even met, who are also struggling, well, it means a lot. **We can do this.**

Today I biked eight miles. But I didn't eat any cabbage.

DIETER'S DELIGHTS & DILEMMAS

_____

_____

_____

_____

_____

_____

_____

_____

_____

February is American Heart month. I'll never forget the time a man slumped over in front of my desk at work.

I remembered my CPR training and quickly began a steady rhythm of heart massage and mouth-to-mouth breathing. Thank goodness the man started breathing before the ambulance arrived. I was so shaken I had to go home. I learned later, however, that the man died in the hospital after saying good-bye to his wife and children.

This month, let's do two things: take a CPR refresher course and get our cholesterol and blood pressure checked. It's part of a healthy life-plan. Bless your heart!

DIETER'S DELIGHTS & DILEMMAS

_____

_____

_____

_____

_____

_____

_____

_____

_____

_____

My mother died at age fifty-seven. Her mother died at age fifty. When I turned fifty-seven I bought myself a new bicycle with a lightweight aluminum frame, shock absorbers, a padded gel-filled seat and a wicker basket.

I plan to ride this bike for at least twenty-five years. A few years ago when my dad was eighty-five, he and I rode fourteen miles on the paved bike path near my home. I love the feeling of being out there on my bike, checking out the scenery, waving to fellow bikers, conversing with my dad. But most of all I'm so thankful that at least half my genes include "bike till you drop" hopefulness.

It's a great way to exercise.

DIETER'S DELIGHTS & DILEMMAS

I f you're like me, you probably show your appreciation to others quite often and consider yourself a good friend.

How good a friend am I to myself? Not very. I am my harshest critic, and I seldom think about showing myself any appreciation. And when I do, it's usually with food. Eating is one way I pamper myself, but now it's the worst thing I can do.

If I'm really going to show myself appreciation and love, I need to do it in healthy, emotionally independent ways. Each week I'm going to designate one day "Self-Appreciation Day" and do something I enjoy with total abandon. This week it's a pedicure while watching my favorite TV show. What's yours?

DIETER'S DELIGHTS & DILEMMAS

_____

_____

_____

_____

_____

_____

_____

_____

_____

_____

FEBRUARY 10

The Girl Scouts are selling cookies! I have a friend who loves Thin Mints, and when she told me she was buying four boxes, my mouth started watering. I seemed to notice Girl Scouts selling cookies everywhere I went. Even coworkers were taking orders on behalf of their daughters.

I want to support a great organization, but I'm committed to *eating better, eating less* and *exercising more*, so I cheerfully "purchased" boxes of my favorite cookies and left the boxes behind.

Every time I got a craving for a cookie I took a quick walk—ten minutes of fresh air and exercise did the trick, and I feel a whole lot better than if I had eaten a box of cookies.

DIETER'S DELIGHTS & DILEMMAS

There are days when we all have a lethargic, down-in-the-dumps, what's-the-use attitude. When the blahs hit, the best fixer-upper is laughter.

Laughter keeps you healthy by building up your immune system and increasing thymus cells that fight viruses. Even fake laughter builds up those cells.

Although she doesn't have a dog, I have a friend who goes to the dog park and watches the dogs frolic with each other when she's feeling down. She gets some exercise walking in the fresh air and always has a good laugh at their playful antics.

Laughter is contagious, so catch some.

DIETER'S DELIGHTS & DILEMMAS

_____

_____

_____

_____

_____

_____

_____

_____

_____

_____

FEBRUARY 12

It's only February and already I feel a bit stressed out by this new healthy-eating/weight-reducing plan. I've got too much to do, there's no sunshine today and yesterday I overate, probably gaining weight instead of losing it.

Then I read about a guy who failed in business, was defeated in numerous public elections including Congress and the Senate. His fiancée died, then he had an unhappy marriage. Three of his four sons died before age eighteen. But finally, in 1860 Abraham Lincoln was elected president of the United States.

Guess I shouldn't give up so easily. Time for a visit to the exercise room and then a nutritious lunch. We can do this!

DIETER'S DELIGHTS & DILEMMAS

_____

_____

_____

_____

_____

_____

_____

_____

_____

_____

D on't you just love how produce departments are providing us with so many good-for-you colorful fresh vegetables that are already washed, cut and ready to pour into salads or cook in the microwave for a quick side dish?

Today, I'm thinking spinach. Yes, those fabulously easy, prewashed bags of fresh baby spinach leaves. I put it in everything: sandwiches, tortillas, scrambled eggs, tossed salads. I toss it into Alfredo or marinara sauce and pour it on pasta. I spread it on a plate to create a tasty doily under deviled eggs or fruit salads. I chop it in tuna and chicken salad. Fresh spinach. It's the bomb. Hard to believe it's so easy and so good for us.

DIETER'S DELIGHTS & DILEMMAS

_____

_____

_____

_____

_____

_____

_____

_____

_____

_____

Happy Valentine's Day. Today let's do something good for our hearts . . . get our blood pressure checked. Many stores and pharmacies offer free blood-pressure checks. I read in a magazine that half of all women over forty-five have untreated high blood pressure. Half! It's scary. Remember, we're on the health train this year, chugging forward, so be good to your heart.

Come on, lace up those walking shoes. Let's go for a heart-healthy walk. Ask a friend to go with you. Or, ask your Valentine. Hold hands. And if we're lucky enough to have a Valentine who will take us out for dinner, bring half of it home for tomorrow's lunch. Portion control, remember?

DIETER'S DELIGHTS & DILEMMAS

_____

_____

_____

_____

_____

_____

_____

_____

_____

I may not be the best eater in the world but my friend Jack is light years behind me and his belly proves it. My favorite thing to do when we're grocery shopping together is to phone Jack from another part of the store and say in a slow, deep voice: "Attention Shopper. Step back, turn around and stay away from the ice cream aisle. Repeat, stay away from the ice cream aisle."

We have a good laugh and go on with our shopping, me in the produce section and Jack in the cookie and chips aisle.

It's hard to lose weight with someone who has chocolate chip cookies in his condo at all times of the day and night. But I'm trying.

DIETER'S DELIGHTS & DILEMMAS

_____

_____

_____

_____

_____

_____

_____

_____

_____

_____

FEBRUARY 16

As a single, self-employed woman I don't have the money to spend on a fancy gym membership. But it doesn't matter since exercising in a skinny leotard, amidst babes and hunks half my age, is a little intimidating.

I know it's terrific for many, but for me, I like the fact that the great outdoors is free. Walking is free. And there's always the wave factor. Leave your house. Walk ten blocks. See how many people you can smile at or wave to. Turn around and walk home. Keep waving. Before you know it you've walked two miles and you feel better than you have all day.

Cost? Zero. New friends? Could be many.

DIETER'S DELIGHTS & DILEMMAS

Unlike me, my mother, Lucy, was never over-weight. Medium build, she wore a size 10–12 and looked good in everything. Her mother, Minta Pearl, was taller, heavier and bigger-boned than I am. So it's in my genes, these size 10 feet, large bones and no doubt the heavy stomach that makes me wonder if I shouldn't buy my blouses in the maternity section.

Today I'm going to stop blaming my grandmother for my bigness. The weight I carry isn't necessary. There are plenty of thin women with size 10 shoes. (My friend Brenda calls my feet *gunboats*.)

No more excuses. It's my body, my life. I can make this work. So can you.

DIETER'S DELIGHTS & DILEMMAS

_____

_____

_____

_____

_____

_____

_____

_____

_____

_____

Remember when we were kids, we were always told to swim with a buddy? It's safer and more fun to swim, hike, snorkel, ski, walk, even shop with a buddy. My sister Catherine and my friends Brenda and Shirley are my fitness buddies.

Catherine walks 10,000 steps a day, according to her pedometer. Shirley will go biking or in-line skating with me on a moment's notice. Brenda, who's trying hard as I am to lose weight, understands every whiny thing I say during our struggle.

Today, let's thank our fitness buddies and remind them how important they are to us. And if you don't have one, get one. Write their names down here.

DIETER'S DELIGHTS & DILEMMAS

So, what do you think? Should we get out the tape measure and record on this page what our measurements are? Sometimes I like the idea because six months later I can measure again and see my progress. Other times the idea is so scary that whenever I see a tape measure I shout, "Be gone!" It's up to you.

Maybe I'll just measure my waist because that's where I store all my gazillion extra calories. It sure would be nice to have a flatter stomach once I start living in that bathing suit.

Meanwhile, let's practice holding our stomachs in. Tightly. Hold it. Strengthen those abdominals. Let's try to hold it in on our fast walks, too.

DIETER'S DELIGHTS & DILEMMAS

_____

_____

_____

_____

_____

_____

_____

_____

_____

_____

I tell myself that I'm not a pet person even though I've had cats, chickens, goldfish, turtles, gerbils, dogs and rabbits.

Now that I'm living alone and don't have kids nagging me to get a pet, I'm content to care for Shirley's two cats whenever she and Wally are away. Strange how cats need the same things I do: a minimum of food (just ½ can for Bubba and ½ can for Boomer), exercise (they'll frolic in the screened-in porch all day) and love. Oh, how those cats love to see me when I arrive each morning.

It's all we really need for good health. A little food, exercise and lots of love.

Are we getting enough of each?

DIETER'S DELIGHTS & DILEMMAS

_____

_____

_____

_____

_____

_____

_____

_____

_____

_____

L esson time. Do we know the difference between physical hunger and emotional hunger? **Physical hunger:** stomach growls and we may feel faint or a little shaky if we've gone too long without food. Five or six small meals a day are better than skipping breakfast and only eating twice a day.

Emotional hunger: we eat because we're sad, stressed, overwhelmed, bored, tired, depressed, angry, tense, fearful, or lonely. Every time we put something in our mouths ask the question, "Am I physically hungry or is this an emotional need?" If it's emotional, find other rewards like a bubble bath, telephone a friend, read a book, go shopping, paint your nails, make something creative, take a drive, watch a movie.

DIETER'S DELIGHTS & DILEMMAS

_____

_____

_____

_____

_____

_____

_____

_____

_____

_____

George Washington was born today in 1732. As the father of our country, he endured political and personal struggles as well as deplorable conditions during wartime.

Thank goodness he didn't give up in times of extreme stress. We're not giving up either. Sometimes it takes superhuman strength to get through the day without overeating or eating the wrong things. Perhaps if we say this five times we can make it through today. *I will not eat the wrong things today. I will only put nutritious foods into my body.*

All right, all right. I'm putting the candy in a box to wrap up for a friend in a nursing home.

DIETER'S DELIGHTS & DILEMMAS

_____

_____

_____

_____

_____

_____

_____

_____

_____

Why are we doing this again? Why are we shifting from candy, cookies, cake, ice cream, chips, white flour, breads, pasta, rice to sensible servings of protein, whole grains, fresh vegetables and fruits? Why? Because we want to look like models? Impress the opposite sex? Fit into a size six? Be the envy of our friends with our stunning new figure?

No. We're doing this because we want to live longer, have more energy, be more confident, have fewer aches and pains, have better health, and so we can finally wear that stunning suit we bought years ago when we were thin.

The rewards are great.

That's why we're doing this.

DIETER'S DELIGHTS & DILEMMAS

_____

_____

_____

_____

_____

_____

_____

_____

_____

_____

Today let's think about what we drink. I've practically eliminated all sodas—diet and regular—from my life. I drink water, tea, milk, fresh-squeezed orange juice (I live in Florida, remember) and an occasional piña colada (once or twice a month).

The sugars and chemicals in sodas do not keep us fit. But water, and plenty of it, does. It took awhile, but I got in the habit of taking a water bottle with me every time I leave the house. Once you become a water drinker you never go back because pure water is, by far, the best thirst quencher. And remember if you're thirsty, you're already dehydrated.

So let's try to drink before we get thirsty.

DIETER'S DELIGHTS & DILEMMAS

_____

_____

_____

_____

_____

_____

_____

_____

_____

_____

I know how I feel some days on this new lifelong health and fitness routine. Discouraged! We all know how important it is to do difficult things with others who can give us support and vice-versa.

So, the minute we feel down, defeated or discouraged, let's call up one of our health-conscious buddies and make plans to do something that involves exercise. And be sure to begin or end that exercise with a hug.

Nothing soothes the human psyche more than a big bear hug. We all need the human touch.

Open up those arms and squeeze.

Ah, I feel better already.

DIETER'S DELIGHTS & DILEMMAS

_____

_____

_____

_____

_____

_____

_____

_____

_____

_____

FEBRUARY 26

Whether we're sitting on a park bench in New York's Central Park, riding a ski lift in Utah, jumping on a cable car in San Francisco, or schooshing down an alpine slide in northern Illinois, we're outdoors, a great place to be. Fresh air, wind, sunshine, blue skies . . . it's all healthy.

Sometimes we get depressed in the winter because of the lack of sunshine, but on a sunny day, we need to get out there, soak it in, be glad we're alive.

Today, if we have a choice to stay in or go out, let's head for the hills and practice our deep breathing while we're out there.

DIETER'S DELIGHTS & DILEMMAS

_____

_____

_____

_____

_____

_____

_____

_____

_____

_____

We know whether we're fat or not, right? Just look at one of those weight/height insurance charts and then weigh yourself. We're fat if we're more than 20 percent heavier than the chart says we should be. Fat is not healthy. But if you're only ten or fifteen pounds within the guidelines (lucky you!) perhaps you're one of those people struggling unnecessarily with your weight.

Is it time to say, "Hey, I don't look so bad. In fact, I look pretty good"? Maybe you need to concentrate on one of the other items in the **SPECIES** list: *Social, Physical, Emotional, Career, Intellectual, Environmental* and *Spiritual*. Time to choose the right challenge.

DIETER'S DELIGHTS & DILEMMAS

_____

_____

_____

_____

_____

_____

_____

_____

_____

_____

FEBRUARY 28

As a writing instructor I try to end all classes that I teach with the words, "Remember, writers write!" Too many times wanna-be writers talk about writing, they read articles in writers' magazines, they attend writers' workshops, but they never get around to actually putting fingers on the keyboard and writing.

Same thing goes for us. *Fitness people get FIT.* We don't just talk about getting fit. We don't keep reading magazines about diet and exercise without putting the pedal to the metal. We don't join weight-loss groups without giving it our all.

Fitness people get fit. Find some stairs. Climb them. I'm doing it. Are you?

DIETER'S DELIGHTS & DILEMMAS

I f this is a leap year, rejoice. It's a gift . . . an extra twenty-four hours to spend as you wish. Actually, every day is a gift. Every single day we have another chance to get closer to being the person we're supposed to become.

God gave us perfect bodies or at least the potential for having perfect bodies. We're the ones who screw them up and cause sickness, disease and early aging by overeating, drinking, smoking, drugs, stress, a sedentary life and environmental poisons.

Today let's leap into a new attitude by taking ownership of our body flaws. Isn't it cool that we also have the potential for fixing our flaws? And it's so simple: *eat better, eat less, exercise more.*

DIETER'S DELIGHTS & DILEMMAS

_____

_____

_____

_____

_____

_____

_____

_____

_____

_____

MONTHLY CHECK-IN

Goals Achieved _____

_____

_____

_____

Triggers Pulled and Buttons Pushed_____

_____

_____

_____

Effective Strategies_____

_____

_____

_____

TALE OF THE TAPE

	Current	Last	Net Loss/Gain
Weight	_____	_____	_____
Hips	_____	_____	_____
Thighs	_____	_____	_____
Arms	_____	_____	_____
Waist	_____	_____	_____
Bust	_____	_____	_____

In 1943, during the middle of World War II, the month of March was declared Red Cross Month by presidential proclamation. Today the Red Cross, in seventy-four countries with a membership of over 100 million, rescues people from flood, tornado, hurricane, fire, earthquake, war and famine.

Hopefully we don't need rescuing from any of those, but we do need to rescue ourselves from a life of bad eating habits, lack of exercise and too much food. Think of the Red Cross today as we struggle to cope with one tiny little disaster after another. Should I eat that cupcake? Take that walk? Have a second helping? Let's be our own Red Cross guardian angels and make this day a success.

DIETER'S DELIGHTS & DILEMMAS

_____

_____

_____

_____

_____

_____

_____

_____

_____

_____

This is serious business, trying to get fit. And the easiest way to fail is to align ourselves with dour, negative, pessimistic whiners. "It's too hard. I can't stick to this eating plan. I hate to exercise! I know if I lose weight I'll just gain it all back again." And on and on.

Friends like that are worse than a room full of germs. What we need are positive people surrounding us this year. Happy people. Friends who encourage us, applaud our successes, make us feel like winners. Even if we only have one e-mail buddy who will help keep us on track, that's success.

Let's write the positive people's names down right here.

DIETER'S DELIGHTS & DILEMMAS

_____

_____

_____

_____

_____

_____

_____

_____

_____

I enjoy watching Tracy sign for the hearing impaired at our church services. I don't understand the language of signing, but when I follow her hands I am overwhelmed with gratitude for the gift of hearing.

On days when I'm feeling down because I haven't watched what I ate or I didn't exercise enough, I try to concentrate on the blessings I have like the gifts of sight, hearing, touch, taste and smell.

At my favorite park when I'm smelling a bright pink rose in full bloom, listening to the birds or touching the cool water in the lake, I feel so blessed that my gloom and doom disappears, and I resolve to have the best body possible.

DIETER'S DELIGHTS & DILEMMAS

MARCH 4

Passing by that tray of donuts or the party tray of meat and cheese is not easy. It takes great strength to say *no thank you* to cookies, candy, ice cream.

Sometimes it takes superhuman strength. Next time we're tempted, think about the ant, that tiny creature that *does* have superhuman strength. An ant can carry twenty times its weight.

In human terms that means if you weigh 150 pounds, you could easily carry 3,000 pounds. Ya, right. Compared to what an ant does, we just have to have a little mental strength to get or stay in shape.

Come on, let's use twenty times our normal mental strength to say no to junk and to eat less today.

DIETER'S DELIGHTS & DILEMMAS

_____

_____

_____

_____

_____

_____

_____

_____

_____

_____

M y friends Brenda and Paul, who joined a national weight-loss group, inspire me to lose weight on my own.

One day they invited me to join them on a nature walk on the mile-long boardwalk that meanders through the woods along a beautiful bay. I forgot my water and was dying of thirst after fifteen minutes on the sunny trail. Without my asking, Paul insisted I take his full water bottle, then shared his wife's bottle with her. What a gift!

Water is so absolutely important for our health. Now I keep water in the trunk of my car and try hard to never, ever leave home without a bottle of H_2O. Are you drinking enough?

DIETER'S DELIGHTS & DILEMMAS

_____

_____

_____

_____

_____

_____

_____

_____

_____

_____

MARCH 6

Whenever I flip channels on TV I'm amazed at how many shopping channels there are. I wonder, *how can so many people spend so much time shopping? Does buying all that stuff make them happy?* Of course not. Stuff, toys, objects do not make us happy. We make ourselves happy, inside and out. If we're happy on the inside with who we are as people, then we can be happy.

If we're happy with our bodies, knowing they're in good shape healthwise, then we can be happy. Check it out. See if you feel happier, more energized and more content when you go to bed tonight after following our simple health plan to the letter today. I know I do.

DIETER'S DELIGHTS & DILEMMAS

It's true, getting into a daily exercise habit can be tough. Especially if we've been couch potatoes for years. But exercise doesn't have to be work. Find something you really enjoy doing and consider it your reward for following through with your food plan for the day. Buy a kayak and explore the backwaters. Try in-line skating. My friend Shirley, who's been skating for years, still enjoys it and she's in her seventies! How about line or square dancing? Take a class. It's a great way to meet new friends as a bonus. Bowling, volleyball, even sex, are all good ways to exercise.

If we do what we love, it'll feel like a reward instead of a chore.

DIETER'S DELIGHTS & DILEMMAS

MARCH 8

I'm meeting so many interesting neighbors now that I'm walking regularly. I'd like to get to know them better. I think I'll make a big pot of "Neighborhood Soup," go for a brisk walk and invite some of them over to my place for a hearty bowl of soup served with a salad.

NEIGHBORHOOD SOUP

Makes 6–8 servings

1 chopped onion
2 cloves garlic
1 tablespoon olive oil
3 (14-ounce) cans low-sodium vegetable broth
2 cups water
6 tablespoons barley
1 bay leaf
1 (28-ounce) can diced or crushed tomatoes (with their juice)
1 cup carrots (halved lengthwise and cut into ¼-inch slices)
1 cup chopped broccoli
1 (10-ounce) package frozen cut green beans
½ teaspoon ea. crumbled dried rosemary and oregano
¼ teaspoon ground black pepper
3 white or red potatoes (cut into bite-size pieces)
1 medium zucchini, (halved lengthwise and cut into ¼-inch slices)
1 (14-ounce) can black beans (drained and rinsed)

1. In a large stockpot, sauté the onion and garlic in the olive oil over medium-high heat until the onions are translucent, about 5 minutes. Add vegetable broth, water, barley and bay leaf. Bring to a boil, cover and lower heat to medium-low; simmer for 1 hour.

2. Add diced or crushed tomatoes with their juice, carrots, broccoli, green beans, rosemary, oregano, salt and pepper. Simmer another 30 minutes.

3. Add potatoes, zucchini and black beans; simmer 30 minutes or longer.

A salesman at the radio station where I wrote thousands of commercials once left a note on my desk: "Pat, you are a gem and a treasure. Thanks for all you do for me and my clients." Those eighteen words stayed on my bulletin board for years. They changed my whole attitude about work. They lifted me up, made me smile, work harder and feel much better about myself.

Do you know someone else who is trying to *eat better, eat less* and *exercise more?* We all do. Let's send that person a note of encouragement today. Remember, we always feel better ourselves when we work hard to make others feel better about themselves.

DIETER'S DELIGHTS & DILEMMAS

_____

_____

_____

_____

_____

_____

_____

_____

_____

_____

Nothing perks up your life more than change. Change is good. Is that why we like to rearrange the furniture, switch around our knickknacks and take trips? It's fun to have different routines and different things to look at in our homes and offices. Change makes us feel invigorated.

Put your hands on your belly. Since we began this adventure on January 1, does your belly feel a little smaller? A little tighter? I hope so! Change in that area is really good. Isn't it fun to slip into a pair of slacks easily that were too tight a few months ago?

Getting rid of that belly fat is a good, good thing, especially for your internal organs.

DIETER'S DELIGHTS & DILEMMAS

_____

_____

_____

_____

_____

_____

_____

_____

_____

My sister Catherine works hard to balance her protein and carbohydrates. She actually eats six smaller-size meals each day. The three extra meals are often healthy snacks that keep her blood sugar at a normal level.

Catherine's favorite healthy snacks include nonfat string cheese, apples or any piece of fresh fruit, peanuts and raisins mixed together, energy bars, fat-free yogurt and shakes made with yogurt, fruit and skim milk.

If we stock up on these items perhaps we won't be so tempted to head for the candy and cookies that might still be lurking in the back of the cupboard.

DIETER'S DELIGHTS & DILEMMAS

Sometimes when we start a fitness plan we get bombarded by the naysayers. You know, all those people—loved ones, friends, neighbors and co-workers—who perhaps don't really want us to lose weight because they like having us as their donut buddy or *let's-go-to-the-big-buffet-for-lunch* buddy or the *let's-order-two-desserts-and-share* buddy.

But we can't let the naysayers pull us into their camp. No! We have to be strong. Write down their names below and let's be careful when we're around them.

Maybe we can love 'em and leave 'em when it's time to eat.

DIETER'S DELIGHTS & DILEMMAS

_____

_____

_____

_____

_____

_____

_____

_____

_____

It's so easy. Unwrap one little chocolate candy kiss. It melts quickly and goes down smoothly. There's a whole dish of them on the table. One more won't hurt. Then another and another. Before you know it a dozen little foil wrappers are scattered. One kiss equals 25 calories. A dozen, 300 calories. If you're on a 1,200-calorie fitness program to lose weight, that's one-fourth of your entire caloric needs for the whole day. And what's worse, you didn't give your body any nutrients . . . just empty sugar and fat calories.

Today's the day we stock up on carrots, celery, bell peppers and fruit.

DIETER'S DELIGHTS & DILEMMAS

_____

_____

_____

_____

_____

_____

_____

_____

_____

_____

MARCH 14

Albert Einstein was born today in 1879. As a man who spent most of his life arguing for international peace, he had a very generous side. In 1944, at age sixty-five, he made a contribution to the war effort by handwriting his 1905 paper on relativity and putting it up for auction. It raised $6 million over sixty years ago!

Today that manuscript is in the Library of Congress. We may never figure out something as powerful as the theory of relativity or do anything that can allow us to donate millions to a worthy cause, but we can live to our potential, physically, mentally and emotionally.

What are we going to do today toward that goal?

DIETER'S DELIGHTS & DILEMMAS

_____

_____

_____

_____

_____

_____

_____

_____

_____

Today is the Ides of March. On March 15, 44 B.C. the Roman ruler Julius Caesar was assassinated. In Shakespeare's play *Julius Caesar,* a soothsayer warns Caesar, "Beware, the Ides of March." But Caesar didn't heed the warning and was murdered. We may not have a soothsayer, but often our bodies warn us of pending problems. March 15 of every year would be a good time for your annual physical, colonoscopy, mammogram or prostate exam.

Listen to your body because it's always your first clue to a serious health problem. Use a red pen to write down any suspicious health problems on the day they occur right here in this book.

DIETER'S DELIGHTS & DILEMMAS

_____

_____

_____

_____

_____

_____

_____

_____

_____

_____

MARCH 16

In 1999 I visited Kuala Lumpur, Malaysia, to attend a wedding. I visited Islamic temples, scorpion, batik and pewter factories, ancient ruins and museums, and saw rubber trees dripping latex. After one long day the tour bus stopped at the foot of the famous Temple Cave. It was pouring rain and none of the other passengers wanted to get out, especially after the driver announced that it was 364 steps to the entrance. I pulled on my jacket and started the climb.

Forty-five minutes and 728 steps later, I'd seen the most amazing cave and holy temple inside a mountain and learned that **we must say yes to all of life's opportunities.**

DIETER'S DELIGHTS & DILEMMAS

_____

_____

_____

_____

_____

_____

_____

_____

_____

_____

As we work to stay on our weight-loss, get-healthy program, perhaps St. Patrick can inspire us. He was actually born in England, sold into slavery in Ireland, turned to religion, then escaped back to Britain.

At age twenty-two, amid great struggle, he returned to Ireland, became a priest, then a bishop and converted many to Christianity. Knowing he faced many obstacles in his life, I like to think of him as a person of great mental strength and determination.

As we face daily battles with our eating and exercise goals, let's remember that St. Patrick never gave up. We won't either. Happy St. Patrick's Day!

DIETER'S DELIGHTS & DILEMMAS

_____

_____

_____

_____

_____

_____

_____

_____

_____

_____

Today I biked seventeen miles. I amazed myself. Granted, it was mostly on drop-dead gorgeous paved paths through my favorite Florida park, zig-zagging around the thick live oaks and palm trees, and around two gorgeous lakes (I only saw one alligator). I wasn't going warp speed. I stopped to rest two times. But I did make it seventeen miles. The point of getting healthy and exercising more is to also enjoy life.

This year let's enjoy our exercising. I love to bike because of the scenery, the friendly people I meet, the birds and other wildlife I see.

Getting in shape also means smelling the flowers and enjoying life to the max.

DIETER'S DELIGHTS & DILEMMAS

_____

_____

_____

_____

_____

_____

M y dear friend Shirley's mom, Clara, is ninety-four years old and lives in an assisted living center. Clara's mind is sharp but her hearing and sight are not very good. She's also a bundle of arthritis with aching joints all over her body. But does Clara sit around complaining? No way. She's up every day, morning, noon and night, walking the halls back and forth, up and down. She tells Shirley, "This is my therapy. I have to walk."

Clara's walking keeps her spirits up and gives her more energy as well. It makes me think, *If Clara can walk every single day, surely I can get out there and exercise four or five times a week.*

DIETER'S DELIGHTS & DILEMMAS

_____

_____

_____

_____

_____

_____

_____

_____

_____

_____

MARCH 20

We inherit all sorts of things from our ancestors. Looks, hair and eye color. Body type. Intelligence. Unfortunately we can inherit a tendency for certain diseases from our relatives as well. Treating the risk factors for disease is the best preventative we can do. Quit smoking. Cut down on alcohol. Reduce your cholesterol. Eat a heart-healthy diet.

Exercise every day. Maintain a positive attitude. Eliminate stress. Laugh. Maybe our generation can be the one to break the cycle and in the future we won't be handing down such things as cancer and heart disease to our children and grandchildren.

DIETER'S DELIGHTS & DILEMMAS

_____

_____

_____

_____

_____

_____

_____

_____

_____

Ever heard the phrase, "Nothing tastes as good as being thin feels"? Even when we lose ten pounds we feel better. Our clothes fit better. We look better. It doesn't require so much effort to bend over. We climb steps easier. Being thin, or thinner, feels terrific. Whether our weight-loss goal is 15 pounds or 150 pounds, each 5-pound loss makes us feel better, happier, proud to put on a smaller size.

Do you remember how that brownie tasted or how you felt when you moved your belt up another notch?

Do you remember that bowl of ice cream or how tall you felt when you looked in the mirror and realized you don't look so wide anymore?

DIETER'S DELIGHTS & DILEMMAS

_____

_____

_____

_____

_____

_____

_____

_____

_____

When you enter the chat rooms of people on a diet, you realize this whole process is about baby steps. One day we watch what we eat, balance our protein and carbs, drink lots of water, run on the treadmill, don't yell at our families. Then the next day we turn into sloths guzzling soda, beer, pizza, chips, candy and whatever else we find in the pantry.

So we take a step back and hopefully tomorrow we can take two giant steps toward success. The important thing is not to beat ourselves up when we slip and fall.

Tomorrow is another day and the road to success begins the minute our feet hit the floor.

One step at a time.

DIETER'S DELIGHTS & DILEMMAS

_____

_____

_____

_____

_____

_____

_____

_____

_____

For the next three days, let's talk about water. No matter how much we weigh, our bodies contain 60–70 percent water. Our blood, muscles, lungs and brains are full of water. Here are six important reasons we must drink water every day:

1. to regulate our body temperature
2. to keep our vital body parts hydrated
3. to aid nutrients in traveling to our organs
4. to transport oxygen to our cells
5. to remove waste
6. to protect our joints and organs

Water is the single most important thing we put in our mouths.

DIETER'S DELIGHTS & DILEMMAS

_____

_____

_____

_____

_____

_____

_____

_____

_____

_____

Many of us don't know how much water we should be drinking every day and unfortunately, most of us don't drink enough H_2O. It's easy to calculate. Take your weight and divide it in half. That's how many ounces of water you need every day. So if you weigh 200 pounds, you need 100 ounces of water or about twelve 8-ounce glasses (or six 16-ounce bottles) of water.

Caffeinated beverages and alcohol actually deplete water from our bodies, so if we drink those we need to drink even more water.

Today, let's take a bottle of water with us whenever we leave the house. They say it takes thirty days to create a habit. Let's begin.

DIETER'S DELIGHTS & DILEMMAS

_____

_____

_____

_____

_____

_____

_____

_____

_____

_____

A s part of our year-long, actually lifelong, fitness plan, we are definitely going to make sure we drink enough water, especially when we exercise. If we're doing hard exercise where we'll be sweating, it's very important to drink extra water.

We should also eat a few salty pretzels before we exercise so we'll have enough sodium to stay in balance. Tap water is perfectly fine for drinking for those of us who live in the United States or Canada.

If we feel nauseated after exercise, have dark yellow urine, a dry, sticky mouth or dry eyes, we are probably dehydrated. Don't let your body get to that point. Drink before, during and after exercise.

DIETER'S DELIGHTS & DILEMMAS

_____

_____

_____

_____

_____

_____

_____

_____

_____

Y ou know it. I know it. Clothes look better on thin people. Thin people can tuck their shirts in and wear belts. Thin women can dress up their waistlines with eye-catching belts, scarves or skinny midriff-showing tank tops.

Today, let's help to motivate ourselves by trying on an old pair of pants that are too small. Write down, here on this page, how many inches you have to go to fit into those pants. Thankfully, one of the first places we lose weight when we start a sensible eating plan is around our middle section.

Let's keep up the good work and we'll be putting on those pants with belts in no time.

DIETER'S DELIGHTS & DILEMMAS

_____

_____

_____

_____

_____

_____

_____

_____

_____

_____

There's an old saying that goes, "I hear, then I forget. I see, then I remember. I do, then I understand." To make something like exercising or eating healthier a habit, we can't just listen to people talk about why we should do it or watch programs on TV that explain the benefits.

We actually have to *do* the action before we can truly understand the benefits. I could spend all day trying to explain how good it feels to snorkel facedown over a coral reef flutter-kicking for hours to keep up with thousands of fish, but until you do it, you'll just never know.

Let's write down the healthy things we want to learn by *doing*.

DIETER'S DELIGHTS & DILEMMAS

_____

_____

_____

_____

_____

_____

_____

_____

_____

MARCH 28

Some people believe in the benefits of fasting; it clears your mind and heightens your senses. Others warn that it can be dangerous for your blood sugar levels.

There is fasting we can do that has no downside:

Fast from anger.

Fast from complaining.

Fast from resentment and bitterness.

Fast from gossip or judging others.

If, for one day, we could fast from all negative feelings or emotions, we would be doing our physical and mental selves a big favor. If we keep reminding ourselves to fast from these negative traits, perhaps we can take up fasting for life.

DIETER'S DELIGHTS & DILEMMAS

_____

_____

_____

_____

_____

_____

_____

_____

_____

_____

We may feel pudgy looking in the mirror because we're not wearing the right clothes. Short or heavy people should not wear horizontal stripes. Taller people with most of their extra weight in the stomach area look great in tops and loose jackets that reach almost to the fingertips. That way the eye slips right past the protruding stomach and down to the hips. We're changing our eating and exercise habits this year. Let's also change our wardrobes. Invite a friend who has a good eye for style and body type to help rework your wardrobe. When clothes help hide our problem areas and enhance our good ones, we feel better, stand taller and have a sense of well-being.

DIETER'S DELIGHTS & DILEMMAS

Sticks and stones may break my bones, but words will never hurt me. It's an old saying, but definitely not true. Reading the words on weight/height charts hurts my feelings. Even though I have forty pounds to lose, the chart says I'm *obese*.

Obese is the most hurtful five-letter word I know. It hurts my feelings and it hurts my health to be obese. If I can just lose five more pounds, I'll slip into the *overweight* category. It's a strange thing. Sometimes the world treats obese people as if they weren't even there. Their bigness makes them almost invisible.

Today I will see them and smile, knowing how they must feel.

DIETER'S DELIGHTS & DILEMMAS

Trying to cut down on my food intake, I made a deal with myself. I call it the *half plan*. If I eat half the sandwich, then I can have a whole apple or peach. If I eat two pancakes instead of four and one piece of bacon instead of two, then I can have half a container of yogurt or a small dish of fruit.

The half plan helps me eat fewer calories while adding more variety to my meals.

Today, try eating half the sandwich or entrée, but then add a few healthy items to your meals. That way, eating half as much can be twice as good.

DIETER'S DELIGHTS & DILEMMAS

_____

_____

_____

_____

_____

_____

_____

_____

_____

_____

MONTHLY CHECK-IN

Goals Achieved _____

_____

_____

_____

Triggers Pulled and Buttons Pushed_____

_____

_____

_____

Effective Strategies_____

_____

_____

_____

TALE OF THE TAPE

	Current	Last	Net Loss/Gain
Weight	_____	_____	_____
Hips	_____	_____	_____
Thighs	_____	_____	_____
Arms	_____	_____	_____
Waist	_____	_____	_____
Bust	_____	_____	_____

L ook back at January 4. Remember how we talked about **SPECIES** and the seven dimensions of wellness? For the next seven days, let's take a close look at each and see how we can incorporate all seven into our health and wellness plan. The first is:

Social—Make some new friends or make plans with your old ones. Nothing helps us stay on track health-wise than choosing friends who are also into keeping their bodies strong and healthy. Plan a healthy dinner for your friends. Take them bowling, skiing, dancing, bike riding, or rent a pool and have a swim party. Our social activities should be less about eating and drinking and more about fun, active adventures.

DIETER'S DELIGHTS & DILEMMAS

_____

_____

_____

_____

_____

_____

_____

_____

_____

_____

*P*hysical—Our physical well-being is mainly what we're concentrating on this year. Think of your body as an office, the shell that holds everything that's going on. Proper diet, nutrition, exercise and well-body checkups at the doctor will keep our offices in top shape so we can get down to the business of being happy, feeling fulfilled, accomplishing our goals, spending time with those we love, being successful in our careers and following our dreams.

None of that is going to happen if we don't take care of the physical part of our beings. So, let's get physical!

Eat better, eat less, exercise more, remember?

DIETER'S DELIGHTS & DILEMMAS

E *motional*—We can expect our emotions to get out of line at various times in our lives. For women, premenstrual tension, pregnancy and menopause can certainly bring on emotional changes. For men and women, emotional ups and downs are caused by stress, pressure at work to produce, tension in relationships, fear of health problems or of loved ones dying, problems at home, and financial worries. What's the big deal about asking for help when you're emotionally exhausted? When your leg is broken you go to a doctor. When your heart or mind is having problems, see a professional therapist, psychologist, psychiatrist, counselor or pastor.

If it's broken, fix it!

DIETER'S DELIGHTS & DILEMMAS

_____

_____

_____

_____

_____

_____

_____

_____

_____

_____

*C*areer—Do you love what you do? Do you do it well? I believe God gives us a special talent to do something well. The main purpose of education is to help us find out what that talent is. If we use it in our career, our work will seem joyful and not a chore.

Who wants to spend eight hours a day hating their job? Work should be fulfilling and rewarding. Reread Martin Luther King Jr.'s quote on January 15 about being a streetsweeper.

If we can't take pride in our work, we're in the wrong line of work. Is today the day we get career counseling? We all should be able to say, "I love what I do!"

DIETER'S DELIGHTS & DILEMMAS

_____

_____

_____

_____

_____

_____

_____

_____

_____

_____

I ntellectual—Lord knows, I'm not a rocket scientist. I've never balanced my checkbook. But I do love learning. I enjoy history, music, art, geography, geology and the human condition. I love to learn new things and about new places. When I'm not exploring, I feel stagnant, like a piece of goo stuck on the floor of life.

That's when I start to plan an adventure or even a one-day, one-tank car trip. This year let's take a class and learn something new. It's never too late. Grandma Moses started painting in her mid-seventies.

Getting healthy means exercising our brains as well as our bodies.

DIETER'S DELIGHTS & DILEMMAS

_____

_____

_____

_____

_____

_____

_____

_____

_____

_____

ON VACATION

*E*nvironmental—This year, as we learn to love our bodies by taking better care of them, we should also try to love the earth and our environment so it will take better care of us. There are ways we can do both.

One way is to walk, bike or take public transportation instead of driving everywhere. Next time we go for a walk, let's get in some good old-fashioned bending exercise by taking along a bag and picking up any trash we see along the way. Bend down, pick it up. Bend down, pick it up. It's great exercise. Good for the waistline and the upper thighs, and great for the neighborhood.

DIETER'S DELIGHTS & DILEMMAS

*S*piritual—Unless you're a scientist, chances are you don't understand the inner workings of the body. But we have faith in our doctors to fix us when something's wrong.

Faith, which is a tremendous gift, is the ability to believe in that which we cannot understand. I don't understand electricity, but I have faith that the light will come on when I flip the switch. I don't understand the problems of the world, but I have faith that God will pull us through.

Faith and spirituality give us hope, carry us through the rough times, help us understand that struggles are good for us and that there is a bright light at the far end of our lives.

DIETER'S DELIGHTS & DILEMMAS

_____

_____

_____

_____

_____

_____

_____

_____

_____

_____

April 8

A great way to work up a good sweat while having fun is dancing. This is one activity the whole family can enjoy. Granted, they may be splitting their sides watching you dance, but who cares? Laughter is good for our overall health too!

Today, let's get in the happy habit of fast dancing. Turn on the radio, find a good rock station or buy CDs of your favorite singers rockin' out. Put on some comfortable clothing and shoes. Stand in front of a mirror, then move those legs, flap those arms, twist that waist, rotate those hips. Jump, shout, wear yourself out! Watch those calories fly away, tiny dancer.

DIETER'S DELIGHTS & DILEMMAS

D id you know that we're not supposed to drink many fluids with our meals? That's because there's acid in our stomach that is used to digest the food, especially proteins. To do the job, the acid has to be at a certain level. If we drink fluids they dilute the acid, which forces the body to produce more acid to get the job done. Therefore, we should drink most of our liquids one hour before meals, or one hour after meals, or in-between meals.

Try drinking your juice midmorning instead of with breakfast. Enjoy a cup of herbal tea with a nutritious midafternoon snack. Remember to take that water bottle with you wherever you go.

DIETER'S DELIGHTS & DILEMMAS

_____

_____

_____

_____

_____

_____

_____

_____

_____

_____

B asically what we all want is to manage our weight and have more energy. The solution is simple. Give your body the fuel it needs at every meal. Whole fruits, vegetables and whole grains digest much slower than juice or refined flour and sugar foods, thus providing more energy that lasts longer. Every meal should also include a small amount of fat and a portion of protein the size of a deck of cards to keep us from feeling hungry a few hours after the meal. Refined foods digest too quickly, making us feel sluggish.

The best energy-producing idea is to have all five food types at every meal: fruits, vegetables, whole grains, protein and fats (nuts, oils, salad dressings).

DIETER'S DELIGHTS & DILEMMAS

What is it about the afterlunch craving for something sweet? How do we satisfy it without blowing our whole program? I want to eat two Snickers, Kit-Kats, Twix or Almond Joy bars. But I eliminated all candy from my house when I gave up candy, cookies and ice cream for Lent. Forty days to cleanse my body of junk. But how do I soothe the sweet-tooth cravings? Sugar-free hot chocolate. Sugar-free root beer. A container of fat-free, sugar-free fruity yogurt. Sugar-free instant pudding is great with a cup of fat-free whipped topping whisked in. Pour it into four or five small wine glasses so when the craving hits, a beautiful parfait is waiting in the refrigerator.

DIETER'S DELIGHTS & DILEMMAS

_____

_____

_____

_____

_____

_____

_____

_____

_____

_____

Today is Big Wind Day. On April 12, 1934, in Mount Washington, New Hampshire, three weathermen observed the strongest natural wind ever recorded on the earth's surface. Gusts reached 231 miles per hour! Speaking of big winds, do you ever wonder if you talk too much, blathering on and on, boring your listeners to death? As we work all year to be better, fitter, more well-rounded human beings, let's work on our social graces. Perhaps we're so consumed with our diet and exercise plan that it's all we talk about.

Today, let's find new subjects to talk about. Better yet, let's put the wind in someone else's sails by listening to what they have to say.

DIETER'S DELIGHTS & DILEMMAS

A diet high in refined sugars and carbohydrates increases our risk of cancer. So can too much alcohol, red meat and fried or fatty foods. Next time we're eating fast food, heaven forbid, let's avoid the chips or French fries that accompany the sandwich. Instead, order a garden salad to accompany that chicken sandwich. We've all heard that people who eat lots of red meat have a much greater chance of getting colon and other cancers. Chicken, fish or soy are better. One or two servings of red meat a week are plenty.

Today, let's cook a chicken breast and slice it on top of a huge garden salad. Soak the chicken strips in tangy Asian fat-free salad dressing. Yummm!

DIETER'S DELIGHTS & DILEMMAS

_____

_____

_____

_____

_____

_____

_____

_____

_____

Having a bad day? Ate too much yesterday? Didn't feel like exercising and now you feel like a schlump? Or maybe one of your appliances broke down? Boss a little crabby?

You think you've got problems. Imagine how the Egyptians felt when the Pharaoh wouldn't let the Israelites leave Egypt. Blight, flies, vermin, frogs, blood, death of the firstborn, darkness, locusts, hail and boils. Now those are serious problems, unlike the things we face.

Let's celebrate each step of our journey of trying to get healthy instead of whining about our little mishaps and failures. Make a list today of all the things you're doing right.

DIETER'S DELIGHTS & DILEMMAS

_____

_____

_____

_____

_____

_____

_____

_____

_____

Today is the holiday for the IRS when all that money to pay for the cost of our federal government comes rolling in. Isn't it funny how we like to bellyache about having to pay taxes?

Yet we sure love to drive on those federal highways, play in the parks and use the services of the government. Sometimes we bellyache about paying the cost to be fit as well. Sure, a loaf of white bread may cost less than a dense, whole-grain bread. A piece of quality fish costs more than a hunk of baloney.

But in the end, it's our bodies we're creating, our way of life, health, longevity. Can we even put a price on that?

DIETER'S DELIGHTS & DILEMMAS

_____

_____

_____

_____

_____

_____

_____

_____

_____

_____

APRIL 16

Go to the store, head right to our favorite section—the produce department—and pick up a bag of those little carrot chips, sliced diagonally and crinkled. Then buy bags of washed and cut celery sticks and broccoli. Put them in a bowl with a few ice cubes in a baggie at the bottom. Leave them next to your chair where you sit at night reading or watching TV and you'll actually eat them. If you buy a bottle of nonfat ranch dressing, or any kind of dressing that suits your fancy and pour a little into a tiny bowl for dipping, you'll finish off those carrots, celery and broccoli in no time.

Congratulations, fiber and vegetable eater!

DIETER'S DELIGHTS & DILEMMAS

_____

_____

_____

_____

_____

_____

_____

_____

_____

_____

Today let's write down the most fun we've ever had exercising. Think back to when you were having a blast and it didn't even seem like a work-out. I remember cross-country skiing over soft hills on a snow-covered golf course. Or the times I've snorkeled in various seas and oceans, kicking my feet with fins on for hours as long as there were fish, sea creatures and coral to watch. Or the day I kayaked, paddling and paddling for three hours, then saw a huge manatee in the water. I jumped out and swam with the gentle giant. Those adventures would all rate an A+ in my exercise book.

What's your favorite, most fun thing to do to work your body?

DIETER'S DELIGHTS & DILEMMAS

_____

_____

_____

_____

_____

_____

_____

_____

_____

_____

APRIL 18

I t's not easy to lose weight. Why? Because we can't just quit eating. Imagine a heroin addict saying he was going to quit the habit by only having one or two hits a day. Wouldn't work. Imagine an alcoholic trying to quit if he was forced to take one or two drinks a day. Well, we who are trying to reduce our weight can't stop eating completely. Every twenty-four hours we must eat three, four, or five times. That's why it's so hard!

We should be awarded a gold medal for every ten pounds we lose because the temptation to eat is always staring us in the face. How strong are we going to be today?

DIETER'S DELIGHTS & DILEMMAS

_____

_____

_____

_____

_____

_____

_____

_____

_____

A clever person once suggested that the seven stages of life are made up of *spills, drills, thrills, bills, ills, pills and wills.* What stage are you in? Personally, I believe that at any age we can be subjected to all or any of the above.

But right now as I try to stay on this fitness plan, I keep falling over, stumbling, backsliding. Then, on the days I **eat better, eat less** and **exercise more,** I experience *thrills* like never before.

Hopefully I won't have any *bills* or *ills* from this experience.

Time for my *pills*—my vitamins and calcium.

DIETER'S DELIGHTS & DILEMMAS

_____

_____

_____

_____

_____

_____

_____

_____

_____

_____

APRIL 20

Those gigan-ta-mundo muffins that some bakeries make that have about 800 calories are out-of-this-world delicious, but oh my goodness, so tough on the calorie counter.

And what's the best part of the muffin? The top of course! These days some bakeries are selling just muffin tops. Yumm. One-third the calories with all the reason we want a muffin in the first place.

If your bakery doesn't make muffin tops, work a deal with your partner. Buy one muffin and split it. Today you get the top and he gets the soft part underneath. Next week you reverse. Everybody's happy. Especially your waistline.

DIETER'S DELIGHTS & DILEMMAS

_____

_____

_____

_____

_____

_____

_____

_____

_____

One year when I was depressed and over-whelmed by all the springtime yard work, my neighbor Coot gave me a lesson in lawn-mower maintenance, then loaned me some gas.

After spending two hours mowing my big lawn, pulling weeds, trimming bushes and hauling brush, I was exhausted physically, but I felt better emotionally than I had in months. There's something about working outdoors that clears the cobwebs and clutter in our brains.

Say, don't those gutters need cleaning? Windows need washing?

DIETER'S DELIGHTS & DILEMMAS

_____

_____

_____

_____

_____

_____

_____

_____

_____

_____

If walking is not your favorite exercise, that's fine. After all, going to the gym puts you in a safe environment, provides you with a great variety of workout machines and is a wonderfully social place.

But if you've tried walking and don't like the solitude or the safety aspect, perhaps you need to adjust your venue, companion or style of walking. Borrow a preschooler from a friend and take him or her for a walk. You'll be chatting away, bending down to examine this and that, sharing stories, skipping to keep up with the wee person, and before you know it you've been around the block a couple of times and it hardly seems like a workout.

DIETER'S DELIGHTS & DILEMMAS

These days cancer strikes without warning and it hits men, women and children of all races, ages, sizes, shapes and backgrounds. But there are so many things we can do to help prevent it from striking us with a deadly blow. If you smoke, stop. If you don't smoke, stay as far away from secondhand smoke as you can get. People have died from secondhand smoke.

Eating whole grains helps reduce cancer risk. *Whole* grains include the germ, bran and endosperm of the grain. Refined grains remove the two most important, the germ and the bran. One report stated that cancer risk can be reduced by 43 percent if you eat whole grains.

DIETER'S DELIGHTS & DILEMMAS

_____

_____

_____

_____

_____

_____

_____

_____

_____

Time for a shake. A nice, rich, thick, chocolate shake, the make-it-yourself-at-home variety. This is the easiest way to get protein and lots of good nutrition into your body.

Start with half a chunk of tofu in the blender. Add a cup or two of skim milk, some protein powder and one carton of fat-free, sugar-free vanilla yogurt. Add a squirt of sugar-free chocolate syrup and a handful of ice cubes. Blend until smooth.

Delicious. It's so good you'll want to keep your blender on the kitchen counter all the time just so you can make these good-for-you, pick-me-up shakes a couple of times a week for snack time.

DIETER'S DELIGHTS & DILEMMAS

One day at work I opened the refrigerator and nearly fainted. It contained seven almost empty ketchup bottles, eight paper bags containing half-eaten lunches, a gallon of fermenting apple juice and numerous slimy vegetables. After tossing nearly everything, I couldn't wait to get home and clean out my own refrigerator. Let's make today National Clean the Refrigerator Day. How old is that mayonnaise and whipped cream, anyway?

Let's buy some colorful plastic baskets to hold more fresh fruits and veggies in our refrigerators. Remember our goal of spending most of our grocery money in the produce department. Think fresh. Fresh, natural whole foods. We're on a mission for life, remember?

DIETER'S DELIGHTS & DILEMMAS

_____

_____

_____

_____

_____

_____

_____

_____

_____

_____

APRIL 26

When a thief stole my mother's jewelry from Dad's house, I felt the grief of her death all over again. The treasures I wanted to pass on to my children were gone. Later I heard them talking about their grandmother . . . how she taught the girls to embroider, took long walks with them, made sweet rolls the boys said were so good you could eat a hundred and the funny games she played with them.

Suddenly I knew I didn't need her jewelry to keep her spirit alive. I could pass on her gentleness, her willingness to always make time for people, her quiet sense of humor.

Being a healthy, fit person means being healthy mentally, emotionally and spiritually as well.

DIETER'S DELIGHTS & DILEMMAS

_____

_____

_____

_____

_____

_____

_____

_____

_____

The amount of food we eat in this country to make one-third of all its citizens overweight or obese is astounding. One doctor said the best way to lose weight is take what we'd normally eat and cut it in half. The easiest way to get in that habit is to start doing that every time we eat in a restaurant. Eat half and pack up the rest to take home for another meal.

The days of *doggy bags* are gone. Now we have *people bags*. Besides, most restaurant meals are much larger than we should be eating. And isn't it nice to have a fully cooked meal waiting for us in the refrigerator the next day?

DIETER'S DELIGHTS & DILEMMAS

_____

_____

_____

_____

_____

_____

_____

_____

_____

_____

APRIL 28

We're supposed to eat only the most nutritious foods from all six food groups every single day to be healthy. Here's a handy reminder:

1. fats, oils, sweets (tiny amounts)
2. milk, yogurt, cheese (2–3 servings)
3. meat, fish, beans, eggs, nuts (2–3 servings)
4. vegetables (3–5 servings)
5. fruits (3–5 servings)
6. breads, cereal, rice, pasta (6–11 servings)

We don't need much, if any, extra fat in our diets. Plus, a serving is a small thing. Think small. Think how you'll look in that swimsuit.

DIETER'S DELIGHTS & DILEMMAS

_____

_____

_____

_____

D o you feel that when the weekend comes you naturally fall off your good-eating health plan simply because your daily routine changes so much? It's a good thing to change our routines, but this weekend remember the lyrics, "Do a little dance, make a little love, get down tonight!" All that means is that we can have fun, get plenty of exercise, get out there, move, groove, shake it up, baby, and make our weekends times of great exercise.

Take the dog for an extra-long walk. Hike to the park and swing on the swings. Enjoy the weekend, but just make sure you incorporate at least thirty minutes to an hour of exercise. Be creative. Do a little dance. . . .

DIETER'S DELIGHTS & DILEMMAS

_____

_____

_____

_____

_____

_____

_____

_____

_____

_____

You know how during the middle of the day or an hour or two after supper we wander into the kitchen, hungry for something, but we're not sure what it is, but we think it should be something crunchy or sweet?

I found it and it's good for us! One of my favorite midafternoon or evening snacks is a half-cup of fruit-flavored nonfat yogurt mixed with a quarter cup of granola. It's crunchy, sweet, creamy, fruity, filling and delicious. Best of all, it's only about 150 calories.

Remember, if we're eating smaller portions at our three main meals, we can have three nutritious snacks every day as well.

DIETER'S DELIGHTS & DILEMMAS

_____

_____

_____

_____

_____

_____

_____

_____

_____

After spending three minutes looking at a fashion magazine, 70 percent of women said they felt depressed, guilty and shameful. Well no wonder! The models in those magazines are all airbrushed to look perfect. In real life none of them, or us, are perfect. Thank goodness.

What I treasure most about the way we look is that we are all unique. No other person in the entire world looks exactly like you. Since none of us are airbrushed in real life, the best thing we can do to improve our looks is to improve our health.

Give yourself that healthy glow, rosy cheeks, great skin, energy and positive attitude by eating a healthier diet and exercising today.

DIETER'S DELIGHTS & DILEMMAS

MAY 2

The word **PLEASE** is a great thing to remember when trying to get fit. Just remember P=*positive statements.* L=*limits.* E=*express emotions.* A=*acceptance.* S=*sense of humor.* E=*encouragement.*

Every morning give yourself a **positive statement** like, "Today, because I deserve it, I'm going to stay with the plan and eat sensible portions of good-for-me food."

Set expanded **limits** for exercising. **Express your emotions** with your best friend. **Accept** your successes or failures and go on. Develop a **sense of humor** about your body and its little flaws. **Encourage** yourself and anyone in your life who is also trying to get fit and stay healthy. *PLEASE*. Do it for you.

DIETER'S DELIGHTS & DILEMMAS

_____

_____

_____

_____

_____

_____

_____

_____

_____

_____

D o you ever wish you could shut off the hunger thermostat in your body? Sometimes I eat when I'm not hungry for various emotional reasons, but most often I feel those hunger pangs.

I try to think about the millions of people worldwide who feel hunger and don't have enough to eat. The sad part is that there is enough wheat, rice and other grains to give every human in the world 3,500 calories a day. It's the world's governments and economy that keep people hungry.

Next time I feel those hunger pangs, I'm going to count my blessings instead of the number of foods I can eat.

Let's write down five favorite blessings below.

DIETER'S DELIGHTS & DILEMMAS

_____

_____

_____

_____

_____

_____

_____

_____

_____

_____

MAY 4

Ever try the cabbage soup diet? Whoa, now there's a plan that gets old really fast. What about the grapefruit diet? That one gives me canker sores just thinking about it. How about the all-protein diet? That'll mess up your digestive system in a big hurry.

Fad diets that restrict you to certain foods should be avoided like a tub full of fire ants. Instead let's work together to choose healthy calorie-controlled or portion-controlled foods rich in fruits, vegetables and whole grains and moderate in dairy, protein and fats.

It's the simplest plan ever. Eat the right kinds of food. Just don't eat as much as you did in your past life. And exercise your butt off. Literally.

DIETER'S DELIGHTS & DILEMMAS

_____

_____

_____

_____

_____

_____

_____

_____

_____

_____

Here are a few facts to help you have a great day eating-wise and health-wise. The average woman in America weighs 144 pounds and wears size twelve or fourteen clothes. That means that for every thousand women who weigh less than 144 pounds, there are a thousand who weigh more. One of every four college-aged women has an eating disorder. Young women aged eighteen to twenty-two are generally stuck on trying to look like those fashion magazine models. It's an unholy goal, one that causes perfectly beautiful, healthy women to stop eating or to eat and purge.

A truly beautiful woman is not a skinny wisp that could blow down in a stiff wind. Set a realistic goal.

DIETER'S DELIGHTS & DILEMMAS

_____

_____

_____

_____

_____

_____

_____

_____

_____

_____

Did you know that three out of every four people do not exercise enough to make their hearts healthy? Are you one of them?

One study said that four groups, especially, do not exercise enough to be heart healthy. They are: African-American women, people with little formal education, the overweight and the elderly.

Yikes. If you're an older, overweight, black woman who didn't graduate from high school, you're in trouble. Time to get serious about this plan for life. Even if you're just overweight, it's time to get serious. Think about it. We're all born with the capacity for good health and slim, trim bodies.

Why do we screw it up?

DIETER'S DELIGHTS & DILEMMAS

_____

_____

_____

_____

_____

_____

_____

_____

_____

_____

Have you tried on last year's swimming suit? Mine feels like I'm trying to stuff ten pounds of flour into a five-pound bag. I hate those rolls of fat around my middle.

So many of us have the belly-fat problem. Makes me feel like I have a barrel for a figure. We swimmers have to bite the bullet and wear that bathing suit, belly fat and all, or we have to start some daily exercises to firm up that area. And there's a bonus! Any exercise you do, even sit-ups to squelch that belly, will improve your cholesterol, lower blood pressure, raise energy level, help you sleep better and, of course, lose weight.

Sit-ups! One, two, three . . .

DIETER'S DELIGHTS & DILEMMAS

MAY 8

Some of us are creatures of habit. We find a form of exercise we love and stick to it, doing the same 5-mile run or the same forty-minute floor routine day after day after day.

Not me. I like variety. Maybe today I'll try out a hula-hoop, sign up for line dancing class or do yoga.

Ever wonder what form of exercise has the highest success rate? The answer is walking, probably because it's free, easy and convenient. We can walk from the time we're toddlers until we're pushing walkers in front of us in old age. We don't need special equipment or clothing, and walking is low impact so there's little or no risk to bones, joints or muscles.

DIETER'S DELIGHTS & DILEMMAS

_____

_____

_____

_____

_____

_____

_____

_____

_____

A unt Bernadine had three favorite words of advice that she said to me many times, "Just say no." Then she'd elaborate: *Just say no* to drugs and smoking. *Just say no* to stereotypes . . . be your own person. *Just say no* to brutality, emotional and physical abuse, violence and cruelty. *Just say no* to ethnic jokes and racial slurs. *Just say no* to doing half the job. *Just say no* to going too fast, whether in relationships or in a car. *Just say no* to wasting time.

Let's add a few more:

>*Just say no* to that supersize burger and fries.
>*Just say no* to that triple-size hot fudge brownie.
>*Just say no* to skipping daily exercise.

DIETER'S DELIGHTS & DILEMMAS

_____

_____

_____

_____

_____

_____

_____

_____

_____

_____

Yesterday, I swam thirty-eight lengths of the junior-Olympic-sized pool across the street. Today, I did fifty lengths only because I wanted to beat my old record.

When we keep track of our exercising it's fun to try to outdo ourselves. Maybe you're going to jump rope for five minutes every day. Then one day you up that to seven minutes.

Start with fifteen minutes on the treadmill and before long you'll be doing forty-five minutes.

Challenge yourself!

DIETER'S DELIGHTS & DILEMMAS

_____

_____

_____

_____

_____

_____

_____

_____

_____

L et's write down a few things that we've been doing right this year when it comes to diet and exercise. Be specific. Here are mine:

I cut out most sweets and when I eat them I try to eat half as much as I used to.

I exercise at least five days a week.

I buy only whole-grain breads, cereals and pastas.

I made friends with Brenda who is also trying hard to lose weight.

From now on I will get an annual physical and have a heart-to-heart talk with my doctor about my health and fitness.

I will always bring half of my restaurant meals home for another day.

DIETER'S DELIGHTS & DILEMMAS

_____

_____

_____

_____

_____

_____

_____

_____

_____

_____

In a study among thousands of Americans, when asked to define their past week in one word, most people answered *stressful* or *hectic*. It's a sad commentary on American life.

It's the high-stress life—too many commitments, activities, organizations, responsibilities, meetings, homework and family life—that keep us going ninety miles an hour.

Today, try to find an hour when you just do nothing. Just sit. Find a bench in a park or a chair on the deck or a step on the front stoop and just sit. Listen to the sounds in your world. Relax. Enjoy a cup of tea or glass of cold water. Take a few deep breaths.

Close your eyes. Tension gone?

DIETER'S DELIGHTS & DILEMMAS

B etween the ages of two and four, 95 percent of all children are highly creative. By age seven, only 4 percent of all children are highly creative. How does that happen? Adults constantly tell children, "Don't do this, don't do that, color between the lines, stand here, sit there, play with these toys." The freedom to be creative all but disappears.

Today, let's figure out a few supercreative ways to stay on track. Take the brownies and cut them into one-inch pieces and freeze them, limiting our intake to one piece a day. Take an exercise mat outdoors and do some free-form exercises under the springtime sky. Wear an especially bright color. Draw flowers on the driveway in chalk.

DIETER'S DELIGHTS & DILEMMAS

_____

_____

_____

_____

_____

_____

_____

_____

_____

_____

I sn't it fabulous when you look at the scale and you've actually lost a few pounds? Time for a reward!

When I lost a few I bought a new swimsuit and didn't feel like the Goodyear blimp when I tried it on. That makes up for the days when everything seems to fall apart and I eat like a woolly mammoth.

When we realize some of the flab is missing, and we have more energy and the courage to try on a new bathing suit, it makes all these months of trying to learn new habits worthwhile. Flowers are blooming. It's time for us to bloom with gusto and grace.

Tell someone today why you are a happy person.

DIETER'S DELIGHTS & DILEMMAS

_____

_____

_____

_____

_____

_____

_____

_____

_____

_____

READER/CUSTOMER CARE SURVEY

HEFM

We care about your opinions! Please take a moment to fill out our online Reader Survey at **http://survey.hcibooks.com**. As a **"THANK YOU"** you will receive a **VALUABLE INSTANT COUPON** towards future book purchases as well as a **SPECIAL GIFT** available only online! Or, you may mail this card back to us and we will send you a copy of our exciting catalog with your valuable coupon inside.

First Name _____ MI. _____ Last Name _____

Address _____

State _____ Zip _____ City _____ Email _____

1. Gender	**4. Annual**	**6. Marital Status**
❑ Female ❑ Male	**Household Income**	❑ Single
	❑ under $25,000	❑ Married
2. Age	❑ $25,000 - $34,999	❑ Divorced
❑ 8 or younger	❑ $35,000 - $49,999	❑ Widowed
❑ 9-12 ❑ 13-16	❑ $50,000 - $74,999	
❑ 17-20 ❑ 21-30	❑ over $75,000	**Comments**
❑ 31+		
	5. What are the	
3. Did you receive	**ages of the children**	
this book as a gift?	**living in your house?**	
❑ Yes ❑ No	❑ 0 - 14 ❑ 15+	

BUSINESS REPLY MAIL

FIRST-CLASS MAIL   PERMIT NO 45   DEERFIELD BEACH, FL

POSTAGE WILL BE PAID BY ADDRESSEE

Health Communications, Inc.
3201 SW 15th Street
Deerfield Beach FL 33442-9875

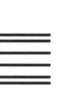

Some days I feel like an overstuffed, weak-willed, overweight, unattractive food monger who doesn't have a brain when it comes to sensible eating.

Did you know that negative thoughts and feelings like these actually destroy our resolve and make it harder to stay on the plan the next day? Negative thoughts breed more negative thoughts. That's why it's so important to stay motivated, upbeat, determined. It's important to surround ourselves with positive people and positive activities that will help us through the tough times.

It's time to become optimistic people, the kind other people love to be around.

DIETER'S DELIGHTS & DILEMMAS

_____

_____

_____

_____

_____

_____

_____

_____

_____

_____

The 4-H organization provides leadership, citizenship and life skills for young people across America and the world. The four Hs are **heart, health, head** and **hands.**

Today, let's think about those 4-Hs in terms of our new lifestyle changes. If we stay on our plan, we're doing great things for our **heart**. Our overall **health** will be improved greatly. Our **heads** are in motion because we're learning new things about life, self-love and the world of good nutrition and exercise. Our **hands** are busy buying and cooking nutritious foods and writing in this book every day.

We are 4-H'ers in spirit. Keep up the good work!

DIETER'S DELIGHTS & DILEMMAS

_____

_____

_____

_____

_____

_____

_____

_____

_____

_____

Calories are energy producers. Losing weight, gaining weight or maintaining weight depends on one simple scientific fact . . . whether or not we are using up all the calories we put into our bodies.

Calories give our bodies the fuel to expend energy. In other words, the amount of physical activity determines how much of the caloric fuel we use up. If we don't use up all the calories, it's stored as fat for the next time we need energy to do something active, but perhaps we don't have the amount of new calories we need. Thirty-five hundred excess calories equals one pound of stored fat. Simple theory. Calories in, energy out.

Now get busy. Move that body.

DIETER'S DELIGHTS & DILEMMAS

_____

_____

_____

_____

_____

_____

_____

_____

_____

_____

Did you know that you lose ninety calories an hour just sleeping? You can lose 114 calories an hour playing cards or writing a letter. Of course if you really want to lose weight, you'll take up something a little more exciting.

Golf, if you walk and carry your own clubs, takes off 324 calories an hour. Think about it. Four and a half hours of golf and you've used up 1,458 calories!

Aerobic dancing takes a whopping 546 calories out of your energy safe. A vigorous swim takes over 500 calories an hour. If you cross-country ski for three hours, you'll use up 2,070 calories, more calories than you may be consuming all day, a surefire way to lose weight.

DIETER'S DELIGHTS & DILEMMAS

_____

_____

_____

_____

_____

_____

_____

_____

_____

_____

Years ago I interviewed Tom Trebelhorn, the manager of the Milwaukee Brewers baseball team after a twelve-game losing streak. I asked him, "How can you keep going after such a downslide?"

He smiled and said, "The Ten-Day Plan. If there's any way a problem will change or go away in ten days I don't waste precious time worrying about it. Most problems get better or go away in ten days."

That means if we screw up with our weight loss/life fitness plan, we shouldn't waste precious time worrying about it.

If we stay on track *today* and every day in the future, that entire pizza, pan of brownies or quart of ice cream we ate will be gone and forgotten.

DIETER'S DELIGHTS & DILEMMAS

Do you have a dream? Is there something you think might be impossible in your life, but you're still dreaming about it? A promotion at work? An exciting vacation to a distant place? A long weekend by yourself in a cabin on a lake?

Treat your dream the same way we've approached this *eat better, eat less, exercise more* plan this year. Gather your faith, believe that you can do it, then make a plan.

Write a letter or do the first thing that needs to be done to make your dream achievable. Do one thing toward your goal every day.

Let's be like the little engine that said, "I think I can, I think I can."

DIETER'S DELIGHTS & DILEMMAS

_____

_____

_____

_____

_____

_____

_____

_____

_____

_____

L eo carried this poem in his wallet for over fifty years before he shared it with me in the early 1980s. I hope it'll change your life as it has mine. It's titled *Only One Minute* (author unknown).

I have only just a minute. There's only sixty seconds in it. I didn't seek it. I didn't choose it. Forced upon me, I must use it. Just a tiny little minute. But eternity is in it.

Think about what we can do with just one minute. Twenty-five sit-ups. A quick back rub for someone you love. Write a list of healthy foods to buy tomorrow. Stand up and touch your toes twenty times.

Just a tiny little minute . . .

DIETER'S DELIGHTS & DILEMMAS

_____

_____

_____

_____

_____

_____

_____

_____

_____

_____

Today is National Maritime Day. I've always lived within a mile or so of a body of water—rivers, creeks, park lagoons, Lake Michigan, and now the Gulf of Mexico and the Intracoastal Waterway.

Somehow, water calms my nerves, brightens my spirit and soothes my soul. I'm happiest when I'm near or in the water.

Today, let's be thankful for the good, clean, plentiful supply of water we are blessed with in this country. Are you drinking enough water?

Remember, our water bottle should be our best friend, going with us every time we leave the house.

DIETER'S DELIGHTS & DILEMMAS

_____

_____

_____

_____

_____

_____

         _____

         _____

         _____

         _____

W hat was your favorite childhood sweet treat? Mine were those marshmallow and coconut-covered snowball cupcakes.

Today, I saw a box at the grocery store for the first time in years and bought it . . . six individual snowballs. In the parking lot I opened one and put myself into marshmallow-coconut, cream-filled, chocolate-cake ecstasy. My plans for healthy eating all but disappeared. I wanted to eat another but at home I put the remaining five in the freezer. After they were frozen, I took them out, cut each into four equal quarters and refroze them. Now when I need a bite of something sweet, I eat one quarter of one snowball . . . 42 calories. My sweet tooth is satiated, and my fitness plan is salvaged.

DIETER'S DELIGHTS & DILEMMAS

Whether you call it perspiration or old-fashioned sweat, it's good for us. When we can work up a sweat when we're exercising we know we're breathing hard and helping our hearts to pump better.

When we strengthen our hearts, it gives us more energy and as an added bonus it helps us look and feel our very best. It's important to start any activity that's going to make us sweat with a warm-up to stretch our muscles. Then have a blast . . . run, skate, bike, dance, ski, jump rope, fast walk, do gymnastics or anything that makes you sweat. When finished, be sure to cool down gradually with more stretching.

Sweat? You bet!

DIETER'S DELIGHTS & DILEMMAS

_____

_____

_____

_____

_____

_____

_____

_____

_____

R ecent studies have shown that the harder the exercise, the more beneficial it is for our hearts. For instance, if we run, swim or do heavy gardening, we can reduce the risk of a stroke by 26 percent. But if we do more moderate exercise like biking, walking or horseback riding, we only reduce the risk of stroke by 14 percent. So perhaps we need to get on the treadmill or into that pool or start digging in the garden at least once or twice a week.

All of it—any exercise—will help keep us fit and help burn calories, but if the risk of stroke is a family concern, consider something a little more vigorous.

DIETER'S DELIGHTS & DILEMMAS

It's time to plant our garden. Even though many of us don't own a speck of dirt, we can still plant this garden.

Four rows of peas: *presence, promptness, preparation* and *perseverance.* Four rows of lettuce: *Let us obey rules. Let us be true to our obligations. Let us be faithful. Let us be loyal.* Three rows of squash. *Squash discouragement, squash indifference, squash criticism.*

Now, reread those last lines and think about how they relate to our diet and exercise plan. Let's use that garden to make our bodies grow and become strong, slim, trim and fit.

Watch that garden grow!

DIETER'S DELIGHTS & DILEMMAS

_____

_____

_____

_____

_____

_____

_____

_____

_____

_____

Next time you start blaming everyone around you for your failures, remember this story about four people named **everybody, somebody, anybody** and **nobody**.

There was an important job to be done so *everybody* was sure *somebody* would do it. *Anybody* could have done it, but *nobody* did it. *Somebody* got angry about that because it was *everybody's* job. *Everybody* thought *anybody* could do it, but *nobody* realized that *everybody* wouldn't do it. It ended up that *everybody* blamed *somebody* when *nobody* did what *anybody* could have done. Moral: *eating better, eating less* and *exercising more* is your job and nobody else's. You and only you are responsible for your health and fitness.

DIETER'S DELIGHTS & DILEMMAS

_____

_____

_____

_____

_____

_____

_____

_____

_____

_____

Obesity, or being considerably overweight, means four strikes against you. All four of these things lead to heart disease.

1. Obesity increases your heart's workload. Get out the tape measure. If a woman's waist circumference is thirty-five inches or more she is more likely to develop heart disease.
2. Obesity raises your blood pressure.
3. It can spike your cholesterol levels.
4. It raises your triglyceride levels.

Think about it. How many diseases can you cure just by changing your eating habits and exercise routine?

You're the one in control here.

You hold the key to a healthy heart.

DIETER'S DELIGHTS & DILEMMAS

_____

_____

_____

_____

_____

_____

_____

_____

_____

_____

When my friends Brenda and Paul joined a group to lose weight before their son's wedding, I decided to kick my own weight loss program into high gear. But they had each other for moral support.

I live alone, and there's nobody but me to offer encouragement late at night when I'm desperate for something salty, chewy or sweet. I felt a little jealous then remembered my weight loss program is mine, not theirs. It's my nutritional eating plan. My daily exercise.

Since evenings are my downfall, I made a deal with myself. I can have a late-night snack as long as it's nutritious.

Tonight it's celery sticks and peanut butter.

DIETER'S DELIGHTS & DILEMMAS

_____

_____

_____

_____

_____

_____

_____

_____

_____

Today is Memorial Day, the day we honor our loved ones who have died. Today might be a good day to talk to the oldest members of your family. Grandparents, aunts, uncles, great-grandparents, the matriarchs and patriarchs. Ask them about your other ancestors. How long did they live? Were they healthy? What did they die from? Make notes. Discover which diseases run in your clan. Then get on the Internet and learn all you can about those diseases. Make notes. Ask your doctor if you're at risk for any of those health problems.

Today, when we remember the dead, let's do something positive to keep the rest of us healthy, fit and living life to the fullest.

DIETER'S DELIGHTS & DILEMMAS

"Hi, how are you?" "Fine, thanks. How are you?" "Fine." How many times have we had that conversation? It's mindless! Since we're in the midst of what we hope is our most life-changing adventure—losing weight, getting healthy—let's share our good news.

The next time someone asks "How are you?" Tell them you're doing terrific! Explain how you've been changing your eating habits since January, exercising more and that you feel better than ever—that you've lost ten pounds! Don't be surprised if they want to know more and ask you to share your tips.

If we open up a bit we might be able to help someone else start to have a healthier lifestyle.

DIETER'S DELIGHTS & DILEMMAS

_____

_____

_____

_____

_____

_____

_____

_____

_____

_____

MONTHLY CHECK-IN

Goals Achieved _____

_____

_____

_____

Triggers Pulled and Buttons Pushed_____

_____

_____

_____

Effective Strategies_____

_____

_____

_____

TALE OF THE TAPE

	Current	Last	Net Loss/Gain
Weight	_____	_____	_____
Hips	_____	_____	_____
Thighs	_____	_____	_____
Arms	_____	_____	_____
Waist	_____	_____	_____
Bust	_____	_____	_____

A dry-erase board has always had a prominent place in my home. Filled with messages, reminders and appointments, it keeps me on top of things. Sometimes I'll write myself a note. *Carrots, not candy!* Or, *Ten days until the reunion. Stay on track!*

Writing encouraging notes to yourself on a dry-erase board is a good way to keep your family informed of your steely determination. They'll see how serious you are about your weight-loss program, and they'll be more inclined to help you. Writing things down for your loved ones is also a wonderful way to communicate. You might even write, "Thanks, dear, for helping me avoid the ice cream."

DIETER'S DELIGHTS & DILEMMAS

_____

_____

_____

_____

_____

_____

_____

_____

_____

_____

JUNE 2

I'm one of those frugal people who often finds a financial excuse not to do something. Join a gym? *It costs too much.* Buy a good bicycle? *It costs too much.* Join a weight-loss group? *It costs too much.*

One day a friend dumped a huge can of reality right at my feet. "How much do you think it costs for five days in the hospital because of a clogged artery? How much does the medication cost for high cholesterol and high blood pressure?" Suddenly that new bicycle didn't seem so expensive. Neither did that aerobics class at the gym.

Are you cutting down the forest to save one tree? Spend a little and you'll get a lot in return.

DIETER'S DELIGHTS & DILEMMAS

_____

_____

_____

_____

_____

_____

_____

_____

_____

_____

My life was one big *hurry*. I hurried to take the children to games, music lessons and the orthodontist, then shopping so I could hurry home to fix supper. My head, back and neck ached, and my whole body felt tense.

Then one day I purchased a white rope hammock on impulse. My son Michael helped me mount hooks into two huge trees. After our inaugural rest, my other three kids took turns with me in the hammock, sharing parts of their day. I felt my eyes close and realized I was totally relaxed for the first time in months. Is it time for you to get a hammock?

The first step to good health is to unwind.

DIETER'S DELIGHTS & DILEMMAS

JUNE 4

Today let's make a list of our blessings, a gratitude list. Write it here, but also type it on a nice piece of paper and attach it to your bathroom mirror. Then, whenever we get discouraged about anything, we can look at that list and wonder how we ever let discouragement become part of our lives.

Let's start: A good strong body. Family and friends who love us. Enough food on the table. A good healthy eating plan. A place to live. Activities and work to keep us busy. Dreams and ambitions. Places to volunteer to make other's lives better. Enough income to live a reasonably comfortable lifestyle. Politicians willing to help run our towns, states and country. Faith.

DIETER'S DELIGHTS & DILEMMAS

_____

_____

_____

_____

_____

_____

_____

_____

_____

_____

Time to reorganize the food in our refrigerators. If you have kids or a spouse who do not need to lose weight, put their desserts and other tempting foods in the back of the refrigerator.

Keep raw fruits and vegetables out in front, the first thing you see when you open the door. That will help remind you to eat them up before they spoil. Wash and cut some of them for easy retrieval when the hungries hit.

Another refrigerator tip is to put your leftovers in individual serving containers so you won't be tempted to eat the whole thing in one sitting.

Also, try freezing bananas, grapes and orange slices for a sweet treat on a hot summer day.

DIETER'S DELIGHTS & DILEMMAS

JUNE 6

My daughter-in-law Amy, a busy nurse and mother of three, is the size of a peanut. Small-boned and petite, every inch of her is muscle and high-powered energy. She runs four to six miles with four friends from the neighborhood three or four times a week at 6:00 A.M. They got so conditioned that some of them swam, biked and ran in a triathlon one year.

Most of us will never exercise to that extent or compete in marathons, let alone triathlons. Even Amy admits her favorite part of running is doing it with friends, the camaraderie she experiences.

Is today the day we ask a friend to join us when we exercise?

DIETER'S DELIGHTS & DILEMMAS

_____

_____

_____

_____

_____

_____

_____

_____

_____

Being overweight is like having an illness or a disease. Carrying extra weight, whether ten pounds or 200 is not how our bodies were designed to function. Think of a race car that is trimmed down with no extra chrome, glass, metal, wood, steel, upholstery, carpet or plastic. Everything on that race car is there for a good reason, and anything else is only holding it back. It's designed for speed, and any extra weight would only slow down that magnificent machine.

Our bodies are the same. Extra weight slows us down and adds strain to our backs and joints, especially our knees and hips. Today, think of yourself like a fine-tuned, sleek race car. Stay on track!

DIETER'S DELIGHTS & DILEMMAS

_____

_____

_____

_____

_____

_____

_____

_____

_____

Today is trading day. Trade in high-fat foods for low-fat or better yet, nonfat foods. Trade in whole milk for low-fat or nonfat milk.

Trade in fatty, red meat for more chicken, fish or low-fat pork. Trade in pastrami, baloney and other sandwich meats for low-fat turkey breast.

Trade in high-fat salad dressings for low-fat or nonfat ones. Trade in milk chocolate for dark chocolate, and eat that sparingly.

Trade in artery-clogging foods for high-fiber fruits and vegetables that will course through your veins and vessels like water sliding down the downspout.

DIETER'S DELIGHTS & DILEMMAS

I admit it, I'm a nonsmoking snob. I get bronchitis when I'm around secondhand smoke, and my health is more important to me than a possible relationship with someone who could potentially damage my health.

Did you know that each puff of smoke causes your heart to pump faster and your blood pressure to increase temporarily? One puff also causes clumping and stickiness in the blood vessels that lead to your heart.

This year we're trying to get healthy physically, mentally, emotionally, spiritually. If you're a smoker, re-evaluate how smoking is damaging all those areas of your life.

DIETER'S DELIGHTS & DILEMMAS

JUNE 10

Anger is often the result of hurt, fear or frustration. It's also possible to feel anger when we're hungry.

If you let your blood sugar drop to an unhealthy level by not eating regular meals and nutritious snacks each day, you can upset your ability to think rationally. Angry feelings may emerge. You might even lash out at someone you love. I've been around people who get very irritable when they're hungry. It's not fun. Many people get shaky and even get a headache if their blood sugar drops too low. If you get cranky or angry when you're hungry, make sure you have healthy snacks in your car, purse, briefcase, desk, office, bicycle basket—everywhere you go.

DIETER'S DELIGHTS & DILEMMAS

_____

_____

_____

_____

_____

_____

_____

_____

_____

When you're serving dinner tonight, wow your family with a few produce facts. For instance, a red bell pepper has twice as much vitamin C as an orange. A sweet potato has twice the recommended daily allowance of vitamin A. The more colorful a vegetable, the more vitamin A it has. Lima beans have seven times more fiber than green beans. A large, baked potato has twice as much potassium as a medium banana.

Get to know that produce department of yours. Research the Internet about how good raw or fresh, cooked vegetables are for you. Make your goal this year to eat more of them and to introduce more fresh veggies to your family.

DIETER'S DELIGHTS & DILEMMAS

_____

_____

_____

_____

_____

_____

_____

_____

_____

_____

JUNE 12

What do we all have but when we give it away it makes us happy and when we get it back, we're even happier? I'm *smiling* here, just thinking how contagious it is.

Yes, a *smile* can turn a crabby diet day into a fun one. If someone upsets you, smile at them instead of showing anger. Smiling is a magic wand. Even when you're alone something good happens when you smile. It's an automatic mood lifter. Try it. A sincere ear-to-ear grin can help keep you on track.

Life is good! We're getting thin and fit and that's a lot to smile about!

DIETER'S DELIGHTS & DILEMMAS

Modern technology makes life easier. Dishwashers, washing machines, electric can openers, power steering. Trouble is, we need the exercise that came from the labor we used to do.

That's why we must find other ways to use up the caloric energy our food provides or it's going to turn into fat. We can do easy exercises like biking five miles per hour, which burns 174 calories in an hour, or we can really push those pedals and go thirteen miles per hour and burn 612 calories in an hour. Walking two miles per hour burns 198 calories. Jogging six miles an hour burns 654 calories. And biking, walking, skating and swimming are more fun than doing dishes or laundry!

DIETER'S DELIGHTS & DILEMMAS

This quote, by Paul Dudley White, is taped to my kitchen cabinet: *A vigorous walk will do more good for an unhappy, but otherwise healthy, adult than all the medicine and psychology in the world.*

I was a single parent of four who lived in a state where I had no relatives to help me with the monumental job of parenting.

I learned that a vigorous walk kept me sane, allowed me to think before I spoke, gave me time to plan and reflect on those busy days when there were three teenagers, a nine-year-old and me all going in a dozen different directions. My walks, often with my dear friend Betsy, kept me healthy enough to parent four kids alone.

DIETER'S DELIGHTS & DILEMMAS

_____

_____

_____

_____

_____

_____

_____

_____

_____

_____

In a survey, Americans gave these excuses for not exercising: They don't have the time. They don't have the willpower. They don't feel like it. A medical reason keeps them from exercising. They don't have enough energy. Here are seven reasons people who do exercise do it every day.

> *It makes them feel better physically and mentally.*
> *It relaxes them, and they sleep better.*
> *It improves their concentration, self-image and their ability to cope with pressure and stress.*
> *It makes them more productive.*
> *It makes them more creative.*
> *It gives them more energy.*

Which group do you belong to?

DIETER'S DELIGHTS & DILEMMAS

_____

_____

_____

_____

_____

_____

_____

_____

_____

_____

Time to play the "what if" game. What if I lose all the weight I want? How will my life change? What if I don't reach my goal? What if I can't keep the weight off once I lose it?

We need to understand one thing. *This is not a diet.* This is a lifestyle change. This is you and me getting healthier, fitter, thinner, having more energy, more confidence and more fun in life. This is not the year of the diet. This is the year we began our lifestyle change. This is the year we began to get healthy in seven ways.

Remember what they are?

SPECIES. *Social, Physical, Emotional, Career, Intellectual, Environmental* and *Spiritual*.

DIETER'S DELIGHTS & DILEMMAS

_____

_____

_____

_____

_____

_____

_____

_____

_____

_____

Time to visit the dollar store. Buy a batch of small plastic containers for leftovers. It helps to get in the habit of putting extra food away in the refrigerator instead of eating that last cup of spaghetti and meatballs or that last serving of mashed potatoes and pork loin.

With the help of toaster ovens and microwaves, it's so easy to reheat leftovers, and I can't think of one food that doesn't taste just as good the second time around as it did the first.

Use those little microwaveable food savers and make a new habit: no more second helpings or finishing food still on the stove. Save it and enjoy not cooking tomorrow or the next day.

DIETER'S DELIGHTS & DILEMMAS

_____

_____

_____

_____

_____

_____

_____

_____

_____

Next time you're at the grocery store, write down the names of five of your favorite cereals. Then write down the number of calories each contains per serving. Also write down the amount of dietary fiber per serving.

Once you see it in print, it's easy to choose the healthiest cereal. You'll probably find that plain oatmeal is the best thing for our health and fitness plan.

I like to take a whole box of instant or regular oatmeal, pour it in a large bowl, add a cup of chopped nuts, a cup of raisins, a couple tablespoons of cinnamon and half a cup of brown sugar. Stir thoroughly and store in airtight containers.

DIETER'S DELIGHTS & DILEMMAS

_____

_____

_____

_____

_____

_____

_____

_____

_____

_____

E ven in the summertime, soup is a delicious, nutritious way to get our servings of vegetables. Sometimes I start with a can of healthy store-bought soup and add the leftover vegetables from the refrigerator. Or I add a big bag of frozen mixed vegetables.

If you have a large family, stretch your budget by adding water and beef or chicken stock, and a little instant rice tossed in after it starts to boil. It's easy to be a creative cook when you're making soup. Don't forget the cabbage and onions. They add fabulous flavor to soup, in addition to providing more vitamins and nutrients. A serving of soup is ten ounces . . . a little less than the amount in a soda can.

DIETER'S DELIGHTS & DILEMMAS

_____

_____

_____

_____

_____

_____

_____

_____

_____

JUNE 20

This is our year to decide: are we winners or losers? A loser is always part of the problem. A winner is always part of the solution. A loser says, "It may be possible, but it's too difficult." A winner says, "It may be difficult, but it's possible." A loser says, "That's not my job." A winner says, "Let me help you." A loser always has an excuse. A winner always has a plan.

Decide today. Winner or loser? Then choose good-for-you foods. Cut your portion sizes down to the recommended amounts. Get out there and move your body enough to work up a sweat. By the end of this year you won't even recognize your beautiful, healthy self.

DIETER'S DELIGHTS & DILEMMAS

_____

_____

_____

_____

_____

_____

_____

_____

_____

_____

There are foods and there are fluids. But, amazingly, milk is both . . . a foo-id. Milk is nutritious and satisfying because it contains protein. Think about it. We humans are created to survive on milk and milk alone when we're born for the first year or so of our lives, whether mother's breastmilk or formula milk. But just because we graduate to solid foods doesn't mean we should give up milk and milk *products altogether.*

To continue to have strong bones we need three servings of milk or dairy products a day. Don't forget to look for low-fat or fat-free daily products. Once you've weaned yourself off whole milk or 2%, you'll never be able to taste the difference. Enjoy that foo-id!

DIETER'S DELIGHTS & DILEMMAS

_____

_____

_____

_____

_____

_____

_____

_____

_____

_____

Today let's work on our intellectual pursuits, specifically our creativity. All of us have the ability to be creative. We may not all be artists, but we can all come up with creative solutions to problems. Here are three easy ways to let that creative energy begin to flow.

1. Sit alone in silence for thirty minutes with no interruptions in a quiet place. Ideas will come.
2. Count down from fifty to one, then meditate for fifteen minutes. More ideas will come.
3. Surround yourself with nature. Take a walk in a quiet park or visit a body of water. Hike in the woods. When relaxing in nature, creative solutions will come for your most serious problems.

DIETER'S DELIGHTS & DILEMMAS

Anne Clark competed in more than 500 running races worldwide and won over thirty trophies. Amazingly, Anne didn't start running until she was sixty-nine years old, and at eighty-seven was still running races. She said that running cured her age-related aches and pains.

If Anne can do that starting at age sixty-nine, think what we can do at our age! It just proves that it's never too late to start to exercise. If you've fallen off the exercise wagon recently, start gradually—perhaps an easy one-mile walk around the neighborhood or on a treadmill. Each day add a few more steps, blocks or miles to your routine, until you, too, can say that all your aches and pains are gone.

DIETER'S DELIGHTS & DILEMMAS

A billion is a difficult number to comprehend, but one ad agency put it into perspective. A billion seconds ago it was 1959. A billion hours ago our ancestors were living in the Stone Age.

We may not be able to comprehend how big a billion is, but we sure can figure out how many pounds we need to lose to be healthy and how many months it'll take to get there.

A safe rate of losing weight is about two pounds a week or eight pounds a month. If you need to lose forty pounds it should take around five months, assuming you stay on track.

Eighty pounds will take the better part of a year. Don't give up!

DIETER'S DELIGHTS & DILEMMAS

_____

_____

_____

_____

_____

_____

_____

_____

_____

_____

I magine a secluded island where the water temperature is eighty-three degrees, the sun shines every day and you're enjoying a massage and a facial on the beach, then swimming in the azure-blue water.

We can't go there every week, but we can take two or three mini-vacations every day. Close your eyes, plant your feet flat on the floor, put your hands in your lap and think about those ocean waves. Listen to the surf. Imagine warm sand between your toes. Take a deep breath through your nose, allowing your belly to expand. Hold it for fifteen seconds. Release your breath slowly. Your blood pressure is no doubt lower than it was a minute ago.

Prescription: three one-minute vacations a day.

DIETER'S DELIGHTS & DILEMMAS

Let's review. We're supposed to eat two to three servings of protein a day. Two to three servings of dairy a day. Six to eleven servings of carbohydrates. Two to four servings of fruits and three to five servings of vegetables. Fats, oils and sweets, use sparingly.

If we add that all up, it's approximately twenty servings of food. If a serving is generally half a cup, that means we can have approximately ten full cups of food a day. Sometimes just knowing how much is enough or too much helps us to stay on track.

At this rate we could eat two cups of food at four meals a day, plus a cup of snack food twice a day.

DIETER'S DELIGHTS & DILEMMAS

_____

_____

_____

_____

_____

_____

_____

_____

_____

G ot the mid-day munchies or the watching-TV snack attack? Hey, it's okay. Snacking is good for you! The diet gurus used to say "no snacking between those three square meals a day" but now nutritionists know that to keep our metabolism moving, having five or six small meals a day makes more sense.

Just stock up on *healthy* snacks. Aim for a balanced combination of protein, carbs, healthy fats, fruits and vegetables. One of my favorite snacks is half a cup of granola mixed in with 4 ounces of yogurt. It's protein, carbs, dairy, fruit and nuts all rolled into one energy-producing snack.

Delicious!

DIETER'S DELIGHTS & DILEMMAS

_____

_____

_____

_____

_____

_____

_____

_____

_____

_____

W e've all heard how important breakfast is. Some nutritionists holler from the rafters, "Eat breakfast! It's your most important meal!" They're right.

One study found that women, especially, who eat breakfast regularly tend to eat fewer calories during the day. In a survey taken by the National Weight Control Registry, they found that 78 percent of its members who had lost and kept off at least thirty pounds ate breakfast every day. After a long night of going without food, your body needs to *break* that *fast* with breakfast.

It gets your metabolism going, gives you energy to work hard, and hey, if it helps us eat fewer calories and keep the weight off, it has to be good.

DIETER'S DELIGHTS & DILEMMAS

_____

_____

_____

_____

_____

_____

_____

_____

_____

D ining out is one of America's favorite pastimes. But when you're trying to lose weight and change lifelong eating habits, sometimes dining out is a deal breaker. Here are five tips for staying on track.

1. Ask for salad dressing on the side.
2. Order entrees broiled, baked, grilled or steamed.
3. Avoid fried items. The oil may not be the healthy kind.
4. Ask the waiter to substitute more vegetables for potatoes, pasta or rice.
5. Ask your server to box up half your entrée before bringing your food to the table.

Bon appetite!

DIETER'S DELIGHTS & DILEMMAS

_____

_____

_____

_____

_____

_____

_____

_____

_____

_____

JUNE 30

Is it time to go shoe shopping? Isn't every day? I'm not talking about four-inch-high stilettos, either. I'm talking about well-made, comfortable, arch-supported, snazzy walking shoes.

Make sure they're very, very comfortable. Go shoe shopping at the end of the day when your feet are as wide and swollen as they ever get. Make sure those walking, running, exercising shoes have plenty of room so you can wiggle your toes.

Don't think for a moment that you can *break them in* if they feel a little tight. Buy a bigger size! Now that you have your proper shoes, lace them up and let the fun begin, happy walker.

DIETER'S DELIGHTS & DILEMMAS

_____

_____

_____

_____

_____

_____

_____

_____

_____

_____

The year is half over. Time for a reality check. Time to memorize the key to making this fitness, weight reduction, health plan work. Here it is:

By **increasing your daily physical activity** and **decreasing the amount of daily calories** you consume, you can **lose excess weight** in the most healthful and efficient way possible.

The great thing about exercising more than we normally have is that daily exercise, for thirty to sixty minutes a day, actually gives us more energy and thus the ability to be more efficient at work and play. Our bodies will work like well-oiled machines when we decrease the calories and increase the exercise.

Turn up the volume!

DIETER'S DELIGHTS & DILEMMAS

_____

_____

_____

_____

_____

_____

_____

_____

_____

_____

JULY 2

For ten years I ran a crash-pad for airline pilots in my home. Once I asked one of the pilots how he remains calm in the cockpit when something mechanical breaks during flight.

He said, **"The Five-Step Plan. 1. Retain control. 2. Define the problem. 3. Review your objectives. 4. Develop and evaluate the alternatives. 5. Decide on a course of action."**

Those five steps can work for us if we fall off our eating plan for life. Say you wolf down an entire bag of chips (the problem). Stay in control. Decide how you're going to avoid chips in the future. Don't buy chips. Course of action? Buy other, nutritious snacks instead. Bingo. Problem solved.

DIETER'S DELIGHTS & DILEMMAS

_____

_____

_____

_____

_____

_____

_____

_____

_____

_____

Sometimes I get discouraged when I just don't feel like exercising at all. I've learned that once you start exercising on a regular basis, your body becomes used to it and the extra energy it gives you makes it easier to do it every day.

However, sometimes your body needs a break just to relax overworked muscles, hence the reason most fitness plans suggest vigorous exercise only three or four times a week. When you're walking, running or working out, if you can't carry on a conversation with someone next to you, you're pushing yourself too hard.

If you can sing, however, you may not be working hard enough. Listen to your body. It's an amazing machine.

DIETER'S DELIGHTS & DILEMMAS

_____

_____

_____

_____

_____

_____

_____

_____

_____

_____

JULY 4

Today is generally a big party/picnic day as we celebrate the independence of our country. Instead of food being 100 percent of the focus, let's make family fun the focus.

Every town in America has a parade. Pack up the folding chairs, grab some water bottles and enjoy the parade. Better yet, bike to the parade route. Afterward, take the family for a swim. Or how about organizing a family softball game?

It's a good idea to make activities the focus of holidays, instead of the food. I, for one, always have such a hard time eating the right kinds of foods and smaller portions at big holiday gatherings.

But today, I'm going to try.

DIETER'S DELIGHTS & DILEMMAS

_____

_____

_____

_____

_____

_____

_____

_____

_____

_____

Ever get annoyed when you're at one end of your house or apartment and you discover you need something at the other end or downstairs or upstairs?

It's time for an attitude adjustment. If you're in the basement and you need something on the second floor, two flights up, take off. Fly up those stairs! Don't pile things at the bottom of the stairs to take up later. Promise yourself from now on, every time you need something or want to put something away, you'll do it right then no matter how far you have to walk or how many steps you have to climb.

That's what fitness is all about. Using energy. Not being lazy. Moving!

DIETER'S DELIGHTS & DILEMMAS

_____

_____

_____

_____

_____

_____

_____

_____

_____

_____

JULY 6

We all eat alone sometimes. Perhaps we're wolfing down that breakfast sandwich from the fast-food place on the way to work. Or eating all the leftovers by ourselves when the kids are spending the night with friends or our spouse is out of town.

Next time you're eating alone, try to imagine that someone, a real nutritionist perhaps, is eating with you. Choose something healthy. Choose a small portion. Balance your proteins, carbs, dairy, vegetables and fruits.

Imagine that the person who's watching you eat loves you and wants you to be healthy, happy and wise.

DIETER'S DELIGHTS & DILEMMAS

_____

_____

_____

_____

_____

_____

_____

_____

_____

_____

I t's been an hour since dinner, but we crave something—anything. Stock up on gum and mints. Often our little cravings come when we think we're hungry and we want to wolf down an entire candy bar or a bag of chips.

But often we're not really hungry, especially if we've been good about eating four to six smaller meals a day.

You could just be thirsty or a little stressed. Popping a mint or a piece of gum in your mouth can help take your mind off eating and help you stay focused on the task at hand.

DIETER'S DELIGHTS & DILEMMAS

_____

_____

_____

_____

_____

_____

_____

_____

_____

_____

JULY 8

Walking on a treadmill is easy and an excellent cardiovascular workout. Here are some tips for first-timers:

1. Start slowly. Gradually increase the speed and/or the incline, work hard for ten to fifteen minutes, then gradually slow it down until you're finished.

2. Keep raising the speed until you work up a good sweat. I worked my way up to three-and-a-half miles an hour.

3. Be sure to bring water. Drink before and after your workout. If you feel really thirsty it is a sign that you're already dehydrated.

4. Wear good walking shoes with support for heels and arches, and comfortable, loose clothing.

DIETER'S DELIGHTS & DILEMMAS

_____

_____

_____

_____

_____

_____

_____

_____

_____

_____

L et's make a list of our weekly accomplishments. Write down all the good things you did this week. Here are mine:

Went to the gym.

Walked three miles, three times.

Skipped dessert and watched portion sizes.

Meditated.

Limited wine to one glass.

Made homemade soup with lots of vegetables.

Ate fruit and fat-free yogurt for snacks.

Did two days of strength training.

Swam thirty minutes twice this week.

Went on two, 10-mile bike rides.

Weighed myself only once this week.

DIETER'S DELIGHTS & DILEMMAS

_____

_____

_____

_____

_____

_____

_____

_____

_____

_____

_____

JULY 10

Did you know that a cup of plain, low-fat yogurt has one-and-a-half times the calcium (needed for building and maintaining strong bones) as a cup of lowfat milk? Plus, yogurt has 60 percent more protein. Yogurt also aids in digestion. When you buy yogurt make sure it says "active cultures" on the label. Our gastrointestinal tracts have over 200 kinds of bacteria in them, so we need the active yeast cultures in yogurt to help maintain a healthy balance in our small and large intestines. Many lactose-intolerant people can still eat yogurt.

All in all, yogurt is one slam-dunk food. Check out some of the new flavors. Sugar-free, fat-free . . . it's time to enjoy.

DIETER'S DELIGHTS & DILEMMAS

Over the last two days I ate a huge brownie, three pieces of cake, a giant cookie, a bacon cheeseburger, greasy fries with ranch dressing, bacon and cheddar cheese loaded on top, plus enough guacamole and chips and Chex mix to serve an entire party.

Why did I do it? I have no idea. But you know what? Today is a new day. Today I got up, had fresh-squeezed orange juice and a bowl of hot oatmeal and then rode eight miles on my bike.

I'm back on track and feeling good. We're going to slip sometimes. It's okay. Beating ourselves up over it serves no purpose as long as we get right back on the health wagon.

DIETER'S DELIGHTS & DILEMMAS

_____

_____

_____

_____

_____

_____

_____

_____

_____

JULY 12

Confession time. I water down the salad dressings. When you think about it, the main purpose of salad dressings is more about wetting the veggies than adding more flavor.

Those vegetables themselves are loaded with flavor, especially the bright colorful ones like red, green, orange and yellow bell peppers, red onions, broccoli and radishes. Even fresh spinach has a distinct flavor.

But when we pour on the salad dressings sometimes we add so many calories and fat that the salad isn't very healthy. So I water it down a bit, use less and my salad still has lots of flavor and a nice, wet, creamy texture.

DIETER'S DELIGHTS & DILEMMAS

_____

_____

_____

_____

_____

_____

_____

_____

_____

_____

Soda companies make enough soda for every man, woman and child in America to drink a gallon a week.

The average twelve-ounce can of soda contains 140 empty calories and ten to twelve teaspoons of sugar! Many people, teens especially, consume six (840 calories) or eight (1,120 calories) cans a day. That's more than half the calories many of us need in a single day.

Empty sugar calories cause weight gain, tooth decay, osteoporosis, even Type 2 diabetes. I gave up soda years ago.

Get those calories from real food.

DIETER'S DELIGHTS & DILEMMAS

_____

_____

_____

_____

_____

_____

_____

_____

_____

_____

Researchers say the average American now has five hours of leisure time a day. I can already hear you groaning over that one, considering our busy, stress-filled lives. But we have machines to do much of our work and quick transportation to get us places faster. So perhaps we do have five hours of leisure time a day. Maybe we just don't use it wisely.

How about an hour for you, an hour for your spouse or significant other, an hour for the kids, an hour for housework and cooking, and an hour for exercise. You might combine time with spouse and kids with the exercise.

Bike riding, hiking or swimming are super family activities. Ready? Let's go.

DIETER'S DELIGHTS & DILEMMAS

_____

_____

_____

_____

_____

_____

July is a great month for picnics. Sometimes the picnic food is good for us, sometimes it isn't. Go easy on chips, dips, white breads, cakes and ice cream.

Grilled meat is good. Fresh fruit and vegetable salads are good. And baked beans are fabulous when it comes to fiber. In fact, baked, black, kidney and pinto beans are among the highest ranking fiber foods with sixteen to nineteen grams of fiber per serving. Other high-fiber foods include cooked peas (thirteen grams of fiber per serving), figs (ten grams) and yams or sweet potatoes (seven grams).

So enjoy the beans at your picnic. Just don't add too much sugar, honey or syrup to the mixture.

DIETER'S DELIGHTS & DILEMMAS

_____

_____

_____

_____

_____

_____

_____

_____

_____

_____

Staying on our eating plan is so worth it when we slip on that swimming suit. When we eat the right foods, eat less of them and get enough exercise, our clothes fit better each week, but it's still hard getting out there in a swimsuit with all that exposed flesh. Just remember this. When you're walking poolside or in the sand along the beach, stand tall, shoulders back, stomach in. Hold your head high and smile at everyone you see. Half of our body image is in the way we project.

It's all about attitude. We are on a mission and we are looking good! Walk tall. And don't forget to go for a swim.

DIETER'S DELIGHTS & DILEMMAS

_____

_____

_____

_____

_____

_____

_____

                                   _____

                                   _____

                                   _____

Sometimes it's hard to eat a nutritious meal every three to four hours like we should when we're trying to lose weight. And it's definitely not a good idea to let your body get hungry, because your blood sugar and energy level drop.

Keep quality nutrition bars in your purse, bag, car, bike basket and backpack. Research the different kinds. Many are actually meal replacement bars. Some are nothing more than glorified candy bars, loaded with sugar and fat. Choose bars that have at least fifteen grams of protein, plus fiber, calcium and folic acid.

Just don't get in the habit of eating these bars instead of a nutritious, well-balanced meal. They're for emergencies only.

DIETER'S DELIGHTS & DILEMMAS

_____

_____

_____

_____

_____

_____

_____

_____

_____

_____

July 18

It's the middle of July. It's hot! An ice-cream bar coated with thick milk chocolate is the only thing I want for lunch. But I'm trying to lose weight so it's time to buy sugar-free frozen treats.

Time to make finger Jell-O. Mix two or three boxes at a time, according to directions on the box, using half the water, and stir into a large cake pan. After it hardens, cut out fun shapes with cookie cutters.

Another cool summer treat is to stir frozen blueberries into a cup of fruit-flavored yogurt.

Buy a cold watermelon and invite the neighbors.

It's true, you can cool off with food. Just keep the calories, sugar and fat to a minimum.

DIETER'S DELIGHTS & DILEMMAS

_____

_____

_____

_____

_____

_____

_____

_____

_____

_____

Just walking from the car or bus to the office in the July heat can use up a lot of your water reserves. If you're a coffee drinker who indulges in a mid-afternoon, pick-me-up, whole-milk latte, you're going to deplete yourself of more precious water because the caffeine in coffee is actually dehydrating. And depending on what you put into that coffee, you could be adding pounds as well.

Try an ice-cold cup of sugar-free lemonade instead. Or iced tea with double the water and half the tea, and a big squeeze of refreshing lemon. Don't let the summer heat mess up your metabolism.

Drink water. Repeat. Drink more water. Carry it with you at all times.

DIETER'S DELIGHTS & DILEMMAS

_____

_____

_____

_____

_____

_____

_____

_____

_____

_____

JULY 20

Sometimes after lunch I get so sleepy I could easily crawl into a corner and doze for an hour. Sometimes it happens after an hour of good aerobic exercise. The yawns. The heavy eyelids. The fuzzy feeling inside my brain.

Why fight it? There is absolutely nothing wrong with a good old-fashioned nap. If you're at work, simply put your head on your desk for fifteen minutes. At home, stretch out in the recliner. Why do you think most South American countries—Spain, Portugal, Mexico, and Italy—enjoy midday siestas?

Our bodies need to refresh and reenergize. A midday nap can give you a couple of extra hours of energy at the end of the day.

DIETER'S DELIGHTS & DILEMMAS

_____

_____

_____

_____

_____

_____

_____

_____

_____

_____

Y ou know how when we first start losing weight we get excited about those styrofoam-like rice cakes because they're so low in calories, but then we quickly grow tired of them and feel like using them for coasters instead of food?

Well, try a little topping. Spoon on a glob of your favorite fat-free yogurt and sprinkle on a variety of berries. It looks like a miniature fruit pizza and is delicious. Or if you have barbecued chicken left over, spoon that on top of the rice cake, sprinkle a little grated cheese and pop in the toaster oven or microwave, just to heat up the chicken.

It takes rice cakes to a whole new level.

DIETER'S DELIGHTS & DILEMMAS

_____

_____

_____

_____

_____

_____

_____

_____

_____

_____

It's time to talk nuts. Pistachio nuts, to be exact. You know, the little green nuts you have to pry out of their shells . . . which is a good thing because it takes longer to eat them and you get fuller faster and feel more satisfied.

Pistachios are a great source of protein, potassium, vitamin E, magnesium, phosphorous, iron and zinc. They help normalize blood pressure and strengthen muscles. Try to get them unsalted for even better health. You can eat forty-nine pistachio nuts (about one ounce) for 165 calories. So start counting those nuts and enjoy a fun snack.

Don't you love the fact that eating properly requires us to have two to three healthy snacks a day?

DIETER'S DELIGHTS & DILEMMAS

To lose weight, 1,800 calories a day is a good goal. Break it down to three 500-calorie meals and three 100-calorie snacks and you'll never feel deprived. Here are ten snacks under 100 calories:

One piece of string cheese and two Wheat Thins
One-half cup nonfat yogurt and a graham cracker
One apple, pear or plum
One slice of turkey on a rye-crisp cracker
One-half cup, low-fat cottage cheese
One-half of a bagel with jelly
One-half of an avocado with salsa
One cup of dry cereal
A rice cake with a teaspoon of peanut butter
Two cups of popcorn

DIETER'S DELIGHTS & DILEMMAS

_____

_____

_____

_____

_____

_____

_____

_____

_____

_____

This weight loss thing is fun! I was craving chocolate, so I just made myself a big dish of warm chocolate pudding. I bought the no-sugar kind and I actually ate two half-cup servings. That's because I wanted *half* of it, not one-fourth. Total calories: sixty. I even added a serving size (two tablespoons) of lite whipped topping, which was only twenty calories.

So for under 100 calories I had a big bowl of warm chocolate pudding that was out-of-this-world delicious. I am now full, satisfied and not feeling a bit guilty because I'm entitled to three 100-calorie snacks every single day. I may have the other half of that pudding, warmed in the microwave, tonight while I'm watching TV.

DIETER'S DELIGHTS & DILEMMAS

_____

_____

_____

_____

_____

_____

_____

_____

_____

_____

I'm still excited about that pudding I made yesterday. So today my snack is lemon chiffon instant pudding. Talk about easy! I poured it into four small wine glasses. What's nicer on a hot summer day than a cold, refreshing, sweet dish of lemon pudding. Buy the sugar-free kind and enjoy two, 4-ounce servings if you want.

Losing weight is not about starving or denying ourselves anything. It's about eating six times a day if we want to and simply watching the serving sizes and the calories in each food. By now we should know exactly what we can eat and how much.

Don't get discouraged if the weight isn't melting off. It's healthier to lose slowly.

DIETER'S DELIGHTS & DILEMMAS

_____

_____

_____

_____

_____

_____

_____

_____

_____

_____

JULY 26

Experts agree, **exercise works** for lowering your risk of cancer, diabetes, high cholesterol, heart disease and obesity. It also works when we're already overweight and we need to get back to normal.

How much do we want to weigh? Aim for the number on the insurance charts. What's your goal for the rest of the year? Can we stay on track and keep doing what we've done all year, or do we need to step things up a bit? Exercise is your best friend when you want to step things up. Choose your favorite sport and do it more often than usual.

Love to golf? Do eighteen holes instead of nine.
Enjoy biking? Ride fifteen miles instead of five.

DIETER'S DELIGHTS & DILEMMAS

_____

_____

_____

_____

_____

_____

_____

_____

_____

_____

Did you know that being overweight probably means we have higher levels of hormones like insulin and estrogen in our bodies than we should? Exercise is the best way to reduce these hormones and lower the risk of certain cancers associated with them. Breast and colon cancer are two. Our gastrointestinal tracts need to be working like a free running drain. The more we exercise, the cleaner our entire GI tract, including stomach, esophagus, and small and large intestines will be. Exercise keeps irritants from lingering too long in the GI spaces and keeps things running on a smooth course.

Don't let your GI gutter get full of chemicals and debris. Clean it out by exercising every day.

DIETER'S DELIGHTS & DILEMMAS

July 28

This time of year it's easy to get plenty of vitamin D from the sun. Not so easy in the winter, especially if you live up north. Twenty minutes a day of sun exposure gives us plenty of vitamin D, although some experts say our bodies lose some of the ability to assimilate the sunshine as we get older. Saltwater fish, egg yolks and vitamin-D-fortified dairy foods also help us get more vitamin D.

So why is this vitamin so important? It helps fight lung cancer, for one. Vitamin D inhibits the growth of tumor vessels and helps prevent the spread of tumor cells.

Isn't it good to learn just why the things we eat are good for us?

DIETER'S DELIGHTS & DILEMMAS

_____
_____
_____
_____
_____
_____
_____
_____
_____
_____

The American Cancer Society warns that a diet high in refined sugar and carbs may increase our risk of breast cancer. A diet high in saturated fats and fried foods leads to obesity and is also a cancer risk.

Today, when we continue our quest to *eat better, eat less* and *exercise more*, know that if they knew how hard we're trying, the American Cancer Society would be proud of us. Our doctors would be proud of us. Our children and parents and brothers and sisters would be proud of us. Let's write down reasons why we're proud of ourselves.

I'm proud of myself for eating cooked oatmeal for breakfast and for going on a long bike ride today.

DIETER'S DELIGHTS & DILEMMAS

_____

_____

_____

_____

_____

_____

_____

_____

_____

_____

JULY 30

Many nutritionists tell us not to eat just before we go to bed, but statistics say that approximately 33 percent of us suffer from insomnia at some point in our lives.

Going to bed hungry may be one cause of tossing and turning once we hit the sheets. One study suggested that eating an oatmeal cookie, a piece of oat bread with a tablespoon of peanut butter or a small bowl of oatmeal is good because oats contain high levels of tryptophan, which can make us sleepy.

I, for one, am a big fan of saving one of my three snacks a day until close to my bedtime. When I do, I sleep like a log in the woodpile.

DIETER'S DELIGHTS & DILEMMAS

_____

_____

_____

_____

_____

_____

_____

_____

_____

_____

Yes! Purdue University researchers discovered a correlation between dairy calcium and losing weight. I've been eating and drinking dairy products all my life, so this is great news.

What they found was that people who consume three to four servings of fat-free milk or milk products like yogurt, cheese and sour cream actually burn more fat than those who only consume one to two servings a day. Mind you, this does not include ice cream, one of our favorite dairy products. Too much sugar and fat in that.

Imagine, drinking three glasses of skim milk a day can actually help us burn fat. So pour on the moo-juice. Try to make it fat-free milk, of course.

DIETER'S DELIGHTS & DILEMMAS

_____

_____

_____

_____

_____

_____

_____

_____

_____

_____

MONTHLY CHECK-IN

Goals Achieved _____

_____

_____

_____

Triggers Pulled and Buttons Pushed_____

_____

_____

_____

Effective Strategies_____

_____

_____

_____

TALE OF THE TAPE

	Current	Last	Net Loss/Gain
Weight	_____	_____	_____
Hips	_____	_____	_____
Thighs	_____	_____	_____
Arms	_____	_____	_____
Waist	_____	_____	_____
Bust	_____	_____	_____

The first day of every month I get excited about my weight-loss program. I weigh myself and rejoice if I weigh less . . . or readjust if it's stayed the same or, heaven forbid, gone up.

One thing's for sure. I'm eating better foods now. I may not be eating small enough portions all the time, but I know I'm healthier overall. If you're discouraged with the numbers on the scale and you've added a whole new exercise regimen to your daily life, know that you may be turning fat into muscle, which is denser than fat.

A square inch of muscle weighs more than a square inch of fat. Is that it, or are the portions still too big? You decide.

DIETER'S DELIGHTS & DILEMMAS

August 2

When I'm in the pool or swimming in the Gulf of Mexico near my home, I'm in heaven. I can do the backstroke, the back crawl, the breaststroke or the sidestroke forever. Especially in salt-water, which makes you so buoyant, the swimming takes on a life of its own. I'm transported to a stress-free world.

The water feels like silk and my mind wanders. Before I know it I've been swimming for a half-hour or maybe even an hour. Twenty minutes of swimming burns 240 calories. So if I swim for an hour I could potentially burn up one-fifth of all the calories I consume on a normal, trying-to-lose-weight day.

What a blessing!

DIETER'S DELIGHTS & DILEMMAS

_____

_____

_____

_____

_____

_____

_____

_____

_____

_____

Got that draggy feeling? No energy? Tired much of the time? Perhaps it's time to start eating power lunches. That includes whole grains, beans, fruits, veggies and protein such as fish, poultry or soy. Protein foods cause a slow, steady blood glucose response that gives us a nice even energy level all morning, afternoon or evening, depending on when the power foods are consumed.

Remember, it has to be whole grains. No white rice, potatoes, pasta or white bread. Think brown foods, not white. Whole grains help us avoid the midafternoon slump that comes from eating white refined carbs.

When we have lots of energy we generally don't overeat. And that's how we lose weight.

DIETER'S DELIGHTS & DILEMMAS

_____

_____

_____

_____

_____

_____

_____

_____

_____

_____

August 4

O vereating is often a matter of trying to soothe cravings. When we don't eat regular meals and regular healthy snacks, those cravings can grow and grow until we dive into the chocolate-covered toffee or eat the whole bag of chips or red licorice.

I'm trying to get in the habit of making my snacks very appealing. Sugar-free pudding served in wine glasses. Or here's a great one. Place an ounce of mixed nuts in one of those cute little Asian sake cups and pop them in the microwave for 20 or 30 seconds until heated. Warm nuts soothe lots of cravings and provide good protein as well. Warm, mixed nuts is also a great idea for party guests.

DIETER'S DELIGHTS & DILEMMAS

_____

_____

_____

_____

_____

_____

_____

_____

_____

This is the season vegetables are fresh, delicious, reasonably priced and available in wonderful colors, shapes and sizes.

So, when you're heading to the beach, pool, camping, kayaking, hiking or any summertime activity, be sure to take the cooler. Stack minibags full of vegetables, fresh from the garden. Toss in some ice packs and add sticks of string cheese, grilled chicken strips, fresh fruit and yogurt.

People eat when they're active so you might as well be the one to provide healthy, beautiful, brightly colored veggies, lean meats and protein-rich daily snacks. That way we can leave the snack wagons alone and avoid the diet-busters like ice cream and chips.

DIETER'S DELIGHTS & DILEMMAS

AUGUST 6

It's tough staying on track to reach our goals, but we can do it. We can do it! Honestly, think how good it feels to lose an inch.

Think how good it feels to suddenly be able to step into our shorts and slacks without leaning on a wall, bed or chest of drawers.

Think how it feels to walk up a flight of steps without huffing.

Think how good we feel after every single exercise.

Even our minds feel better! Moving these grand, glorious bodies of ours makes them work more efficiently and they become stronger, more agile and more beautiful. We can do it. Drop that donut! Forget the thick latte. It feels better being firm, fit and fabulous.

DIETER'S DELIGHTS & DILEMMAS

_____

_____

_____

_____

_____

_____

_____

_____

_____

L osing weight can be stressful. Every day we have to decide what to eat. How much to eat. Is it healthy? Did we exercise enough? We worry when the scale doesn't move down as fast as we'd like. Sometimes we snap at our families or give them dirty looks when they eat ice cream.

Stress raises the levels of cortisol in our bodies. Cortisol is a hormone which can increase our risk for high cholesterol and high blood pressure.

We do not want this new weight loss, healthy eating and exercising adventure to cause us any stress. Breathe deeply. Find fun things to do. Enjoy your family and friends. Meditate. Pray. Write in this journal. Stay calm, serene, happy.

DIETER'S DELIGHTS & DILEMMAS

_____

_____

_____

_____

_____

_____

_____

_____

_____

_____

AUGUST 8

D id you ever hear the saying, "Everybody wants to go to heaven, but nobody wants to die"? I suspect if you're reading this book you have a dream that your heaven on earth has you in tip-top shape, thin, full of energy and taking no drugs for diseases or ailments.

We all want the *heaven-on-earth* healthy feeling but nobody wants to deny themselves their favorite foods. I used to like eating an entire bag of malted-milk balls or five pieces of pizza instead of just one.

But now that I'm into the *eat better, eat less, exercise more* routine, I know I'm not on a diet. I'm into life. Long, happy and healthy.

DIETER'S DELIGHTS & DILEMMAS

_____

_____

_____

_____

_____

_____

_____

_____

_____

Y ou know how they always tell us on an airplane that if there's an emergency, to put our own oxygen mask on first and then our child's or companion's? There's a good reason.

If we don't take care of ourselves first, we can't be any good to anyone else. Same holds true when we're running busy lives, working stressful jobs, raising children, carving out relationships, running homes. If we don't find time for our own nutritious meals, exercise, recreation and plenty of sleep, we can't be good spouses, parents, teachers, workers.

Plus, as an added bonus, if we take care of ourselves first, we then feel great about taking care of others.

Funny how that works.

DIETER'S DELIGHTS & DILEMMAS

August 10

Hopefully we've all lost a few, if not *quite a few*, pounds . . . especially if we started this grand weight loss adventure in January. Chances are, friends, family, co-workers and neighbors are noticing the change.

"Wow, you look like you've lost weight! How'd you do it?" "You must be on a diet. Which one?"

When people notice, it makes all these months of struggle worthwhile. Flash them your biggest smile, whirl around to show off your new-and-improved figure and say, "I'm *eating better, eating less* and *exercising more.*"

Congratulations on sticking with it. Remember, this is not over when we reach our goal weight. It's for life.

DIETER'S DELIGHTS & DILEMMAS

_____

_____

_____

_____

_____

_____

_____

_____

_____

_____

I t's **Triple Triumph Time**. What's that? It's you and me standing in front of our mirror each evening before bed. We think back on our day and think of three different ways we triumphed over temptation, the triple triumph.

"I had a salad and half a sandwich on 100 percent whole grain bread for lunch instead of a cheeseburger and fries. I helped my family understand that this plan is for life for all of us. I walked around the block after supper instead of eating pie a la mode."

What triple triumphs did you have today? Let's do at least three things every day toward reaching our goal of lifetime good health and fitness.

Write them down.

DIETER'S DELIGHTS & DILEMMAS

August 12

Everyone has read those personal ads, people advertising for dates. Of course the ads make the person sound too good to be true.

Mine would be something like, *Fit, fun, feisty, funny middle-age woman loves biking, swimming, snorkeling and socializing.* Of course I'm not as fit as I'm going to be in a few months after I whittle off more of this extra poundage, but I've certainly got the *fitness for life* mentality.

It's important to have good self-esteem. The fact that we're working so hard to get our bodies back the way the creator intended them to be is a good thing.

Today, let's write an ad for ourselves below. Would you want to become friends with you?

DIETER'S DELIGHTS & DILEMMAS

_____

_____

_____

_____

_____

_____

_____

_____

_____

I sn't it hard when your best friend suggests you stop for ice cream? Or your companion at the movie insists on a tub of hot buttered popcorn? Or the tray of high-fat appetizers floats past your nose at a party?

It's maddeningly frustrating because often we don't have the strength to say, "No thanks, I'm really working to get rid of my extra pounds and get healthier." It's hard to say no to friends. But when we always say yes to others, we're really saying no to ourselves.

No, you don't deserve to be thin and feel good in your clothes with better health and more energy. No, you should make others happy, not yourself.

Hey! Wake up!

DIETER'S DELIGHTS & DILEMMAS

_____

_____

_____

_____

_____

_____

_____

_____

_____

_____

As a professional speaker I've learned techniques over the years to quell prespeech butterflies. The best advice I ever received was to leave the room just before I'm introduced, walk fast while saying, "I'm the best speaker they've ever heard. I'm going to knock their socks off! This audience will love me!" It works. Every time I bound up to the podium full of positive energy.

It'll work for us as we lose weight. Instead of being discouraged when we have a setback, stand tall, shoulders back and say, "I'm the strongest willed person I know when it comes to losing weight. I can see my new figure! Today, I will do it and I will do it well!"

DIETER'S DELIGHTS & DILEMMAS

_____

_____

_____

_____

_____

_____

_____

_____

_____

Repeat after me. **I will not be taken in by products, services or claims offered by unscrupulous, fraudulent companies in the** weight-loss industry.

Do you know that the fraudulent weight-loss products and services industry makes over $5 billion a year? Come on, people! No cream, pill, aerosol, copper bracelet, stretchy gizmo or exotic gadget is going to help you lose weight. Once again, it's calories in, energy out.

What you eat must equal your output of energy, otherwise the food is stored as fat. Don't fall for the scams. Use your money to buy nutritious food, instead. Or a membership at the gym.

DIETER'S DELIGHTS & DILEMMAS

_____

_____

_____

_____

_____

_____

_____

_____

_____

_____

We are not alone, especially in America. One-quarter to one-third of all Americans are overweight.

Forty percent of all women and 24 percent of all men are trying to lose weight. Let's get inspired by each other. What's wrong with sitting down next to a heavy person on a bus or plane and starting up a conversation: "I don't know about you, but I've been on about sixteen diets in my lifetime and I'm still struggling. I wish there was an easy answer."

Before you know it, you may be hearing about all sorts of good eating ideas or ways to fit exercise into your daily life.

Lean on others. We're in this together.

DIETER'S DELIGHTS & DILEMMAS

_____

_____

_____

_____

_____

_____

_____

_____

_____

_____

A ristotle said, *We are what we repeatedly do. Excellence then, is not an act, but a habit.* Researchers say it takes thirty days to create a habit and ninety days to break one. So, let's not get discouraged, we can become excellent at getting healthy.

Here's another quote I like from Ralph Waldo Emerson. *Most of the shadows of life are caused by standing on our own sunshine.* Are we sunshine blockers by using negative talk about how we've failed or about how hard it is to change old habits? Instead of, "I can't believe I ate the whole thing," let's say, "Tomorrow and the next day and the next, I'm definitely using portion control. I will succeed!"

DIETER'S DELIGHTS & DILEMMAS

_____

_____

_____

_____

_____

_____

_____

_____

_____

_____

I once ate with a man who had salad, rolls and an enormous plate of spaghetti and meatballs piled three inches high, enough for three people. He finished it and went back to the buffet table for another heaping plate of spaghetti. Pure gluttony.

I'm convinced that portion control is the answer to most overweight problems. Each portion should fit inside your cupped hand or be the size of a deck of cards.

And when looking at the number of calories on the carton, make sure you see how many portions are in the container. It may say 120 calories, but the container holds three portions. That means 360 calories if you eat the whole thing.

DIETER'S DELIGHTS & DILEMMAS

_____

_____

_____

_____

_____

_____

_____

_____

_____

_____

Today, the birthday of America's first pilot, Orville Wright, is National Aviation Day. Flying has become one of America's favorite and safest means of transportation, yet there are many people who have never been up in a plane.

Until you see the earth from the window of an airplane, you never really get a sense of how amazing this planet is.

Sometimes we who are trying to lose weight never get a sense of the big picture either. Write down your weight goal, how you're going to look after you reach that goal, what kind of clothes you're going to buy and how you plan to stay slim, trim and ready for any adventure you can think up.

DIETER'S DELIGHTS & DILEMMAS

_____

_____

_____

_____

_____

_____

_____

_____

_____

_____

AUGUST 20

Craving chocolate? Who doesn't? The *Journal of Food Science* says we don't have to feel totally guilty.

If dark chocolate suits our fancy, it's a good thing. First of all, dark chocolate contains compounds that can actually give us more energy. And it's not just the small amount of caffeine. It's a big dose of antioxidant phytochemicals called flavonols that help push more blood into the brain. That makes us feel more alert.

So perhaps at work part of our midday snack could be a piece of rich, creamy, dark chocolate.

One piece, remember, not the whole bag.

DIETER'S DELIGHTS & DILEMMAS

_____

_____

_____

_____

_____

_____

_____

_____

_____

_____

L isten, love, learn and laugh. I'm so convinced that these words are the backbone of life that I painted them on a ceramic plate and gave it to my cousin Whitney as a wedding gift.

The most important is to laugh. Ethel Barrymore once said, *"You grow up the day you have your first real laugh—at yourself."* When you stumble and go off your eating plan, laugh it off, learn from the mistakes and start fresh in the morning.

When we hear complaints from our family because we're serving more salads and fewer desserts, prance around like a rabbit eating lettuce.

Help your family laugh at the situation and then just keep on making them healthier, as well as yourself.

DIETER'S DELIGHTS & DILEMMAS

_____

_____

_____

_____

_____

_____

_____

_____

_____

_____

AUGUST 22

If you're not getting enough sleep, fix it. Getting enough sleep is the most important thing you can do for your good health.

Studies have shown time and time again that the average adult needs seven to nine hours of sleep a night. Not four, not five, not six. Your body needs good, uninterrupted sleep to function, stay healthy and maintain a disease-fighting immune system.

Pick a bedtime and stick to it. Think you have to fold just one more load of clothes before bed? No, you don't. Readjust the chore list if you're the only one up after bedtime doing housework.

ZZZzzzzzzzzzzzzzzz.

DIETER'S DELIGHTS & DILEMMAS

_____

_____

_____

_____

_____

_____

_____

L ifting weights, for both men and women, is a terrific way to increase muscle strength and density. Every week we should schedule a few weight-lifting sessions. Get professional help to learn the different machines or read up on the proper way to lift hand weights at home. If you feel pain when lifting weights you're probably damaging the muscle.

A great snack to eat after weight lifting is something with low-fat protein and complex carbohydrates. The protein helps repair muscle fibers that are broken down during weight lifting, and the carbs help the protein get to your hungry muscle cells. Try a soft taco or a turkey sandwich on whole grain bread.

DIETER'S DELIGHTS & DILEMMAS

_____

_____

_____

_____

_____

_____

_____

_____

_____

_____

Ever wonder why bananas are shaped like big, bright smiles? Maybe because there's so much to smile about when you eat bananas. Talk about a super snack.

A banana is not only easy to take along anywhere because it comes in its own packaging, it's always clean when you unzip the peel. Unlike other sugary sweets such as candy and cookies, which zap your blood sugar into the red zone very quickly, a banana provides a slower, more steady stream of energy for a number of hours.

A banana contains water and fiber, and it's loaded with vitamins A, C, B_6, and potassium, and it's very easy for the body to digest.

DIETER'S DELIGHTS & DILEMMAS

_____

_____

_____

_____

_____

_____

_____

_____

_____

_____

I knew having a sweet tooth was not good for me, but its temptations were everywhere! Last March I gave up candy, cookies and ice cream for forty days during Lent. I did fine because I discovered how good warm, fat-free, sugar-free chocolate pudding is.

When Easter dawned my sweet tooth had all but disappeared. My body had come to appreciate the slow-releasing carbohydrates from whole grains and fruits. The cravings for high-density sugar and fat were gone.

It's simply a matter of retraining our bodies. They say you can create a habit or major change in thirty days.

Warning: like any addiction, don't fall off the wagon and dig into a bag of chocolates.

DIETER'S DELIGHTS & DILEMMAS

AUGUST 26

For the next four days I'll share four myths and the myth busters that I found in *Health Magazine*.

Myth #1: Brown equals whole grain. *Wrong.* There are so many brown posers out there, companies that add color and other additives to their breads and cereals to make you think they are whole grain. The truth is that unless it says 100 percent whole wheat or whole grain, it probably isn't.

One of the many bonuses in eating whole grains is that they make us feel fuller, longer. Why eat a white-bread sandwich that's going to leave you feeling hungry an hour later, when the rich, whole-grain bread sandwich will keep you feeling full and satisfied for hours?

DIETER'S DELIGHTS & DILEMMAS

_____

_____

_____

_____

_____

_____

_____

Myth #2: Dairy makes us fat. The truth is that cutting dairy defeats our good efforts for weight loss.

Our bodies need dairy products (granted, fat free or low fat are best) to *prevent* weight gain. Eating dairy products daily nearly doubles our efforts at body-fat reduction and weight loss. How? Calcitrol in dairy products helps fat cells convert less sugar to fat. It also helps burn more body fat.

Dairy also helps conserve calcium for stronger bones. All in all, it's best to follow the government's recommended amounts of dairy, which is three to four servings of low- or nonfat dairy products every single day. Good news, eh?

DIETER'S DELIGHTS & DILEMMAS

Myth #3: The more calories we cut, the more weight we'll lose. Truth: If we let our caloric intake fall below 1,200 a day, we actually decrease our metabolism and muscle mass. In other words, too few calories a day will make us tired and lethargic, and our metabolism (the body's engine) slows down drastically. Exercise revs up the metabolism and nutrient-dense foods, not refined foods, pack more vitamins and minerals into fewer calories.

So let's toss the chips, cakes, cookies, candies and anything made with white flour, and make sure we eat at least 1,200 calories a day when we're trying to lose fat inches. Many active adults, especially men, can eat 1,800 calories a day and still lose weight.

DIETER'S DELIGHTS & DILEMMAS

Myth #4: Cutting carbohydrates helps us lose weight. Truth: We need carbs for energy. We need 100–130 grams of carbohydrates a day, not twenty to thirty a day that some popular all-meat-all-the-time diets proclaim.

When you cut back on carbs, yes, you lose weight but only temporarily. What really happens when you cut carbs down to twenty or thirty a day is that fatigue sets in. You become constipated. You become irritable. You run a much greater risk of heart disease and colon cancer. It's not a pretty picture.

We are smarter than that, aren't we? Say it again. We are *eating better, eating less* and *exercising more.*

DIETER'S DELIGHTS & DILEMMAS

_____

_____

_____

_____

_____

_____

_____

_____

_____

_____

Yikes! Some candy companies are adding plant sterols to chocolate candy bars and calling them health foods. Beware, fitness friends, it's a ploy to sucker us in to eating more dense fat and sugar calories than we need. No matter what they add to chocolate candy, the high-sugar calories combined with the amounts of fat in chocolate put these so-called health-food chocolate candy bars at the very teeny tiny tip of the food pyramid.

There are far too many good-for-us foods in the wide, expansive middle and bottom sections of the food pyramid to waste time eating candy bars. Besides, 200 extra calories a day equals a twenty-pound weight gain over a year.

DIETER'S DELIGHTS & DILEMMAS

_____

_____

_____

_____

_____

_____

_____

_____

_____

_____

Half the battle of becoming a fit, thin, healthy person is being aware of the clues that stimulate inappropriate eating. For me, I tend to eat inappropriately in restaurants.

The food is there, somebody else cooked it, I'm hungry so I chow down, often eating too much. Another time is at parties and other social occasions when I'm surrounded by people and conversation. I eat, eat, eat while I talk, talk, talk, often not even realizing how much I'm eating. Same thing happens when I'm alone watching TV at night. I get the munchies.

But now that I know my three weak areas, I'm doing better: I think before I eat.

Write down your weak zones.

DIETER'S DELIGHTS & DILEMMAS

_____

_____

_____

_____

_____

_____

_____

_____

_____

_____

MONTHLY CHECK-IN

Goals Achieved _____

_____

_____

_____

Triggers Pulled and Buttons Pushed _____

_____

_____

_____

Effective Strategies _____

_____

_____

_____

TALE OF THE TAPE

	Current	Last	Net Loss/Gain
Weight	_____	_____	_____
Hips	_____	_____	_____
Thighs	_____	_____	_____
Arms	_____	_____	_____
Waist	_____	_____	_____
Bust	_____	_____	_____

Thanks to *Woman's Day Magazine*, I learned about *swappers*. If I'm craving cookies, I can swap for a small chocolate-chip granola bar. Instead of 280 calories for four sandwich cookies, it's only 190 for the granola bar.

Got the late-night ice cream craving? One-half cup premium ice cream, only four ounces, at 250 calories can be swapped for an entire low-fat ice cream sandwich with only 110 calories.

Craving hot, salty, French fries at 230 calories for a small order? Substitute three-and-a-half cups of light microwave popcorn at only 120 calories.

Remember, 100 extra calories a day adds up to ten pounds of fat on your body per year. Ugh!

DIETER'S DELIGHTS & DILEMMAS

_____

_____

_____

_____

_____

_____

_____

_____

_____

_____

They're insidious. Downright sneaky. Even their name is gruesome. *Trans-fatty acids*. They lurk in prepackaged cookies, cakes, brownies, pastries, breads, even fresh bakery products. They keep foods from turning rancid on grocery shelves. I remember reading about a twinkie that was still in good shape six years after it was made!

Trans-fatty acids are in fast foods, especially fries, chips, doughnuts, and croissants. Trans-fatty acids can raise your cholesterol levels, clog your arteries and make your heart say, "Enough, already!" Trans-fatty acids are the fats that remain solid at room temperature. Surely, we can pass up packaged treats to save our hearts, can't we?

DIETER'S DELIGHTS & DILEMMAS

_____

_____

_____

_____

_____

_____

_____

_____

_____

While buying all those school supplies for the kids, buy yourself a new white board and mount it in the kitchen for all to see.

Today, write a list of five or six healthy snack options for yourself and the kids on the white board. Things like a fruit smoothie made in the blender with fresh fruit, tofu, milk and ice or whole-grain toast with peanut butter. A glass of milk with fruit. Whole-grain cereal and milk. String cheese and whole-grain crackers. Fat-free yogurt.

Having the list on the white board for all to see will help steer you and the kids away from the unhealthy snacks. They may even come up with ideas of their own.

DIETER'S DELIGHTS & DILEMMAS

_____

_____

_____

_____

_____

_____

_____

_____

_____

_____

Back-to-school time can be stressful for everyone in the family. If you're feeling the crunch of having to be in so many places for so many people, remember three words. **Moderation. Moderation. Moderation.**

If you feel your eating plans slipping by the wayside, don't make any sudden promises to "stay off chocolate for life!" Instead, promise yourself a new, moderate lifestyle. Instead of five pieces of rich chocolate, tell yourself you can have one piece a day. Poof! Craving gone.

My sister-in-law eats one of those chocolate calcium chews every morning to help soothe her chocolate cravings. Remember, moderation. It's a full-proof plan.

DIETER'S DELIGHTS & DILEMMAS

_____

_____

_____

_____

_____

_____

_____

_____

_____

After I exercise I'm so hungry I could eat most of what's in the refrigerator and/or cupboards. The trick is to plan ahead.

I stock my purse, gym bag, car or backpack with a few good-for-me, afterexercise pick-me-ups. A cereal bar loaded with fiber and protein is good. Or a healthy whole-grain homemade raisin muffin. A mini-whole-wheat bagel with one ounce of soft cheese or cream cheese.

We need afterexercise snacks to get us over the hump so we don't grab a soda, chips and candy bar out of a vending machine. I've discovered when I eat a healthy snack and drink a bottle of water, I'm good to go for another couple of hours.

DIETER'S DELIGHTS & DILEMMAS

September 6

After a late breakfast at 10:30 A.M., I attended a matinee at 1 P.M., and it was 4 P.M. before I could eat again. By then all I could think of was a huge hot-fudge sundae, which I ate with chocolate peanut-butter ice cream, malt powder and whipped cream. Then I had a fast-food chicken sandwich.

All I can say for myself is that I only had one scoop of ice cream instead of two or three. Granted, had I eaten a healthy sandwich first, I might have ordered sherbet or sorbet. But I'm not beating myself up.

Once every six months we can have hot fudge and ice cream, can't we? Of course! This isn't a diet, remember. It's a lifestyle.

DIETER'S DELIGHTS & DILEMMAS

_____

_____

_____

_____

_____

_____

_____

_____

_____

L osing weight is not an *all-or-nothing* activity. If you eat the whole cake, don't toss your healthy eating plan to the wind and say, "I already blew it so I might as well eat whatever I want."

Get right back on that horse! I've blown it every couple weeks all year. But I get right back up on this healthy lifestyle and try again. One thing that helps me is that I'm not a slave to the scale. I only weigh myself every three or four weeks.

This is not about beating ourselves up.

This is about putting ourselves on a pedestal for every good thing we do to lose and maintain our ideal weight.

DIETER'S DELIGHTS & DILEMMAS

_____

_____

_____

_____

_____

_____

_____

_____

_____

_____

Remember our acronym for the **SPECIES** concept? Those seven key areas of our life also describe the different kinds of hunger we have.

Social: We hunger for friends. *Physical:* The only hunger that needs to be addressed with food. *Emotional:* We often eat because of emotions, but we should find other outlets. *Career:* Eating at work is often just a bad habit because there are donuts in the break room. *Intellectual:* Studying often makes us eat when really we're just hungry for knowledge. *Environmental:* All around us are eating temptations we can resist. *Spiritual:* Yearning for comfort from above may feel like physical hunger. Instead, try praying.

DIETER'S DELIGHTS & DILEMMAS

This is the peak of produce season. Let's celebrate the harvest! Invite your friends over for a community salad party. Make it a block party and invite the whole neighborhood.

Ask them to raid their gardens or visit the local farmer's market and buy one item for a giant salad. One person can bring fresh lettuce or a mixture of greens. Another can bring tomatoes. Check off the list of goodies: cucumbers, mushrooms, carrots, broccoli, cauliflower, onions, radishes, snap peas, celery, zucchini, and red, green, yellow and orange bell peppers.

Ask each person to bring one item (cleaned and ready to toss into the salad), then dump it all into a giant bowl, bring out the salad dressings and dig in.

DIETER'S DELIGHTS & DILEMMAS

At the turn of the twentieth century, life expectancy was around fifty years. Now it's almost up to eighty. Amazingly, America's seniors are mostly healthy, vibrant, energetic folks who don't plan to wind down in retirement, but want to see new things, do new things, explore and live the good life.

If you're in your twenties, thirties, forties or fifties, see what you have to look forward to? If you're a senior, you've arrived. The most important thing is to get there in good health.

Today, promise yourself that you are going to eat right and exercise more so the last half or third of your life can be as much or more fun than the first part.

DIETER'S DELIGHTS & DILEMMAS

_____

_____

_____

_____

_____

_____

_____

_____

_____

September 11 is a day to be thankful that we live in the greatest country in the world, where we have freedom, democracy and a high standard of living.

Most Americans have the luxury of buying machines and gadgets that do much of our work for us, which frees up time for exercise and enjoying good food with our families.

As we pause each year to remember the tragedy on September 11, 2001, let's be mindful to take care of ourselves and our families by feeding these bodies only the most nutritious foods and to exercise our bodies into the best of health. We are strong!

DIETER'S DELIGHTS & DILEMMAS

_____

_____

_____

_____

_____

_____

_____

_____

_____

_____

Sometimes our bodies fool us. We think we're hungry, but we're actually thirsty. Whether we're working in an office job or on our feet in a factory, long work hours can play tricks on our hunger and thirst thermostats.

Drinking lots of water throughout the day, especially at meetings, helps us stay alert. When energy goes down in the midafternoon, our bodies need a protein snack: hard-boiled egg, cheese, nuts or a high-protein energy bar. Soda and a candy bar midafternoon is the worst thing we can do. The sugar load will actually make us more tired. Make a list right here of all the nutritious, high-protein foods to take to work.

DIETER'S DELIGHTS & DILEMMAS

_____

_____

_____

_____

_____

_____

_____

_____

_____

_____

M yth: Water makes us retain fluids and feel bloated. Fact: Salt is the culprit. Water is a natural diuretic. It actually helps flush our system of toxins that, in turn, keeps us healthier.

Eating too much salt—chips, fries, burgers, salted nuts, pretzels—is definitely not good for us. It can cause high blood pressure. And it makes us feel fat and bloated. Our shoes and rings feel tight, our stomach extended.

Today, let's look at all the food labels for sodium content. Three cans of soup in my cupboard contain 33–41 percent of the daily requirement of sodium for one 8-ounce serving. That's why we should limit our canned food consumption. Fresh is best.

DIETER'S DELIGHTS & DILEMMAS

Today let's make a list of our daily health tasks. Get out a big, black marker and print in large letters:

1. Exercise.
2. Wear sunscreen.
3. Eat fresh, raw fruits and vegetables.
4. Sit quietly for ten minutes, meditating.
5. Exercise the brain. Do a puzzle, read or write.
6. Express love, verbally or by action.
7. Pray for someone.

Every few days we should make a new list of daily health tasks.

I sure feel better than I did in January.

Do you?

DIETER'S DELIGHTS & DILEMMAS

_____

_____

_____

_____

_____

_____

_____

_____

I *do not* like how I feel at the end of the day when I've blown it with my eating plan. But I love how I feel the next morning after a whole day of really staying on track.

Are we going to feel bad or are we going to do what's necessary to feel terrific? Here's an assignment for today. Type these words eight times in large bold type: **I CAN DO IT!**

Cut them out and tape them all over your house: on the refrigerator, over the sink, in the snack cupboard, on the bathroom mirror, on the top of your computer, on your desk, on the dashboard of the car, in your office.

Every bit of encouragement helps.

DIETER'S DELIGHTS & DILEMMAS

_____

_____

_____

_____

_____

_____

_____

_____

_____

_____

It doesn't matter when we start our new healthy-for-life eating plan. Perhaps today is your very first day. Here's a tip.

Don't tell everyone about your goal to lose weight and get healthier. Why? Because there are people out there who will not understand our determination to want to change. They will try to undermine our goals. *Aw, come on, you can have just one double cheeseburger and an ice cream.* Only tell those people close to you who will be supportive in every way.

We are vulnerable. Losing weight is not an easy task. Sometimes it feels impossible! So confide in the supporters and let the underminers be surprised next time they see a thinner, healthier you.

DIETER'S DELIGHTS & DILEMMAS

_____

_____

_____

_____

_____

_____

_____

_____

_____

Close your eyes. Take a deep breath and visualize. See yourself thin. Mentally imagine your new, thinner body. See the slimmer hips? No more over-the-top stomach? Why even that flab under your upper arms is gone!

Now imagine your face. Those chubby cheeks are now showing off that stunning bone structure of yours. And those legs! Wow. Muscles where muscles belong. Shapely.

Now, find a photo of you before you gained the weight and put it in plain sight where you'll see it every day. Buy a dress or pair of pants in the size you intend to be after you lose the weight and hang it from the ceiling in your bedroom. Visualize! We can do this!

DIETER'S DELIGHTS & DILEMMAS

_____

_____

_____

_____

_____

_____

_____

_____

_____

SEPTEMBER 18

Hurry up! Faster, faster! We're late! Do you hear those words every day? It's time to push your overload button.

Slow down. Take a deep breath. Relax. If you're always on the go, you're probably one of those people who eat on the run. I bet you even eat standing up sometimes. Do you eat in your car? At your desk?

Personally, I cannot bear to eat standing up. It feels like a breach of protocol, etiquette or good manners. Plus, it's not good physically to eat on the run or standing up.

Eating should be a relaxing, comfortable, slow, social activity. Set the table. Enjoy the food. Make mealtime a happy event. When you eat slowly, you eat less.

DIETER'S DELIGHTS & DILEMMAS

_____

_____

_____

_____

_____

_____

_____

_____

_____

_____

Diversity is one of my favorite words. I love all things different. I love the fact that people come in all different sizes, shapes, colors, backgrounds, religions, educations, and financial means.

Today, let's be mindful that we humans possess many, many different body types. Some have hourglass figures. Some are pear- or apple-shaped. The scientific words are ectomorph, mesomorph and endomorph.

Our bone structure, height, shoulder width and shoe size all help define our body type. We just need to take that basic mold and whittle it down a bit to make it the healthiest specimen we can.

DIETER'S DELIGHTS & DILEMMAS

_____

_____

_____

_____

_____

_____

_____

_____

_____

What inspires you? What helps you find your spiritual self? What raises your level of consciousness? What motivates you? Satisfies your soul? What is it? Your faith? Religion? Reading spiritual books? Other people who seem to have a peace about them? Prayer? Your soul partner? Friends? Mother Nature?

To be completely happy, we need to think about what inspires us to be better human beings and then, of course, we need to use that inspiration to actually become better people. Seeking a level of spirituality is one of our goals this year. Treating our bodies kindly with proper nutrition and exercise is a level of spirituality that will take us the distance.

DIETER'S DELIGHTS & DILEMMAS

L ooking for an exercise that's easy on the joints and produces less stress and less sweat? Think water. Even if you live in the middle of the desert, you can find a swimming pool somewhere. Some hotel pools even offer memberships for local residents.

Water workouts are so good for you. One of the best is walking across the pool for an hour. Check out the new water toys at sporting goods stores. Balls, jugs (or fill up an empty plastic gallon or half-gallon milk jug with water), noodles, water weights and water-exercise DVDs will help you get moving in the water.

For the ultimate in weightlessness with little or no stress on joints, jump in! The water's fine!

DIETER'S DELIGHTS & DILEMMAS

SEPTEMBER 22

September 22, 1903 was the birthday of the ice cream cone. Italian emigrant Italo Marchiony applied for a U.S. patent on the pastry mold he invented to hold his luscious lemon ices.

Next time I'm temped to have a double scoop of rocky road or chocolate marshmallow fudge ripple cashew, I'll ask for the homemade waffle cone with a scoop of lemon ice instead.

Or what about adding a half cup of fresh raspberries to a cup of raspberry-flavored nonfat yogurt in a waffle cone? Fresh strawberries in strawberry yogurt? Blueberries in blueberry yogurt?

Imagine, a healthy cone, one we can enjoy every day at snack time if we like!

DIETER'S DELIGHTS & DILEMMAS

_____

_____

_____

_____

_____

_____

_____

_____

_____

Counting today, there are only 100 days left in this year. One hundred days. Let's start a new habit today and see if, by the end of the year, we can't make it a part of our life forever.

Write the numbers from one to one hundred on your calendar for each day through December 31.

Today, do one stomach crunch in bed before you get up. Tomorrow, do two. The next day, three and so on. By December 31 we'll be doing 100 stomach crunches each morning before we get out of bed.

Once today, twice tomorrow until you're doing 100 by December 31!

DIETER'S DELIGHTS & DILEMMAS

_____

_____

_____

_____

_____

_____

_____

_____

_____

_____

SEPTEMBER 24

It's 4 P.M., dinner's not until six and I'm starving! Honestly, I could eat an entire bag of family-size chips and salsa.

Instead, I filled up my favorite large mug with ice and sugar-free, peach-flavored iced tea. I bought the powdered ice tea mixes and use twice as much water as they call for. Then, I ate half of an eight-ounce container of fat-free, lemon-chiffon yogurt. Total calories seventy, and I'm stuffed.

Amazing what that refreshing glass of iced tea and a little yogurt can do to fill up a stomach. I am so proud of myself for thinking before I eat.

This year I've finally mastered healthy in-between meal snacks. I know I can make this plan last for life.

DIETER'S DELIGHTS & DILEMMAS

Someone once said life is made up of *the tender teens, the teachable twenties, the tireless thirties, the fiery forties, the fretful fifties, the serious sixties, the sacred seventies, the aching eighties, shortening breath, death, sod, God.*

I'd like to think that I can be tender, teachable, tireless, fiery, serious and sacred no matter what age I am. I'm also planning to avoid the fretfulness, the aching and the shortening breath by following my weight loss and daily exercise plan for life.

Good health is a choice. Every single day, every hour for that matter, we have decisions to make. Excuse me. Time for my healthy snack and then a long bike ride. It's a beautiful fall day!

DIETER'S DELIGHTS & DILEMMAS

Sometimes my mouth waters thinking about deep-fried chicken or fish. Or those deep-fried donuts mother used to make. She'd drop spoonfuls of batter into a deep fryer that had six inches of melted fat. But those days are long gone. Now I know that baked, poached, steamed and grilled food tastes just as good and oh boy, is it ever better for us!

Now that we've become sensible cookers, we could just toss out those frying pans. The oven, gas grill, toaster oven and microwaves are our new best friends.

Wouldn't you rather get that teeny, tiny bit of fat or oil in your diet by eating a small piece of chocolate than by eating some fried food?

DIETER'S DELIGHTS & DILEMMAS

Here's a quiz. What three things provide natural healing endorphins that will help boost our immune systems? Give up? Hopefully, you're going to like all three answers. They are **exercise, sex** and **laughter.**

I'd say to be really healthy we need to do at least two of the three every day. Laughter is the easiest. You don't even need to find something funny. Just stand in front of the mirror and start laughing. Even fake laughter builds up healing endorphins and helps us avoid disease and viruses. It's all part of being a well-rounded, healthy human.

When you think about it, sex can incorporate all three—just don't laugh too hard while you're having it!

DIETER'S DELIGHTS & DILEMMAS

Life is hard. You and I both know someone who is suffering right now. Perhaps you are suffering. Please, let's not eat our way through our miseries. There are ways to deal with problems besides eating. Go for a long walk. Meditate. Talk to a friend, pastor, rabbi, minister or counselor. Write about it. Pray about it. Give back. Volunteer. Help someone else who is suffering.

It's amazing how that works. Help someone else and our own miseries often disappear or lessen. So what if you had a bad day? We have a brand new twenty-four hours tomorrow.

Life is hard. Overeating is easy. Deal with life.

Don't trade one problem for another.

DIETER'S DELIGHTS & DILEMMAS

Self-image is about walking tall, feeling proud, having energy. Am I fat, skinny or just right? Am I weak, strong or a combination? Am I smart, dumb or in-between? Am I a good person, bad, likeable, obnoxious, exuberant, shy, friendly, annoying, optimistic or a complainer?

If we tell someone they are a liar, chances are good they will become one. If we tell ourselves we are overweight, weak, stupid, bad, obnoxious or annoying, chances are we will take on some of those qualities.

Today, let's concentrate on our good qualities. We are working hard to get our body weight down to a healthy level. Plus, we are good, helpful, friendly, smart, honest, positive people. Yes we are!

DIETER'S DELIGHTS & DILEMMAS

Fall is a great time for outdoor games. Whether we're into touch football, street hockey, softball, tennis, golf or hoops in front of the garage, we need to prepare by eating a healthy snack before the game. It'll give us energy to finish and will help us lose weight as we burn off calories playing the game.

Try a small handful of dried fruit, like raisins or apricots. Or one slice of whole-grain bread with honey or peanut butter. Two pieces of fresh fruit is a good choice. If the game is really intense, instead of just bringing a water bottle, bring half fruit juice and half water to help maintain blood sugar during the fun.

Let the games begin!

DIETER'S DELIGHTS & DILEMMAS

Sometimes hot, salty, crisp fries are so tempting I find them hard to resist. So try oven fries, made with hardly any fat and therefore much easier on our weight-loss plan. It's as easy to make one serving or enough for the whole family.

Wash baked potatoes and slice lengthwise, leaving the skin on. Put slices on a baking sheet sprayed with non-stick canola or olive oil spray. Lightly spray the potato slices as well. Sprinkle on any spice, Cajun, Indian, Creole, garlic salt, onion . . . be creative. Bake at 450 degrees until golden brown, usually twelve minutes. Turn them over at least once during baking.

And if you want them really crisp, place them under the broiler for a couple minutes. Yum!

DIETER'S DELIGHTS & DILEMMAS

OCTOBER 2

No matter how convincing those TV, radio, Internet and newspaper ads are, there are no supplements, diet pills, magnetic jewelry, body wraps, herbal formulas or diet drink concoctions that will make you lose weight. You may lose a little water weight, which is not healthy by the way, but not fat!

If you like pouring money down the drain instead of cutting back on the wrong kinds of food, go ahead. It's your body, your life, your health. But come on, you're reading this book. You want to get healthier. You want to lose those excess pounds of fat.

You're on the right track. Every day we're a little healthier. Stop kidding yourself; it's work, but we can do it!

DIETER'S DELIGHTS & DILEMMAS

_____

_____

_____

_____

_____

_____

_____

_____

_____

_____

Today let's step outside ourselves and find someone to compliment about their body image. When I was a young girl, my Uncle Jim, an Air Force general, used to tease me about being such a "big girl." My bones and body weight were bigger than any of his four daughters, his wife or my other cousins.

It stayed with me my whole life. I was the *big* girl. Perhaps it was a self-fulfilling prophecy.

Today, let's find a young person we can compliment. To my favorite thirteen-year-old I say, "Hailey, you are so strong and tall, and a great athlete. What a beautiful, healthy body you have!"

DIETER'S DELIGHTS & DILEMMAS

_____

_____

_____

_____

_____

_____

_____

_____

_____

Today, invite your thinnest, healthiest friend to lunch. Watch the way he or she eats. My stepmother Bev has been my role model since 1982 when she married Dad. Bev has never been an ounce overweight in her life.

Now, in her eighties, she's a picture of health, walks every day, bikes, loves to dance. She also loves to bake and is the best cook I know. But she's not big on sweets. Rarely does she eat more than a bite of those incredible cakes, pies and cookies she makes for my father. I rarely see her take second helpings of anything. She enjoys food but eats slowly and when she's full, she's finished.

Who's your eating role model?

DIETER'S DELIGHTS & DILEMMAS

_____

_____

_____

_____

_____

_____

_____

_____

_____

_____

Some days are better than others. But you know what? Every day we wake up, it's a brand new start! A new chance to make this lifestyle plan work.

Today, the minute I feel hungry I'm going to fix a nutritious snack. Let's make today, *stock up on the snacks day.*

Let's stock the refrigerator with fresh fruits, veggies, yogurt, string cheese, sliced turkey and skim milk.

Let's stock our desks or lockers at work with healthy snacks.

Let's put nutritious whole-grain energy bars in our cars, briefcase, backpack or purse.

Let's never be far from a nutritious snack again.

DIETER'S DELIGHTS & DILEMMAS

_____

_____

_____

_____

_____

_____

_____

_____

_____

_____

Two unrelated studies came to very similar conclusions. One was that most people overeat between 7 and 10 P.M.

The other study found that 93 percent of people who watch more than one hour of TV a day are overweight.

TV is a mindless activity—which I love—but I've discovered it is more satisfying if I'm doing something else while I sit there. So I do crafts, mend clothes, open the mail, give myself a manicure or pedicure, write letters, lift weights or read the newspaper during commercials.

Remember, more than one healthy snack is *not* an option during TV time.

DIETER'S DELIGHTS & DILEMMAS

_____

_____

_____

_____

_____

_____

_____

_____

_____

_____

Picture yourself at dinner time. Are you standing at the sink wolfing down last night's leftovers so you can rush out to a meeting? Or are you eating in your car after grabbing a burger at the drive-though? The fact is that it takes fifteen to twenty minutes after you eat until you truly feel satisfied.

Ever notice that very few French women are fat? It's because meals in France are long, luxurious, social occasions. Each course is an exquisite experience with friends and family. Conversation is more important than second helpings. Sit down. Spread a cloth napkin in your lap. Take a deep breath. Eat, talk, enjoy.

Slow down!

DIETER'S DELIGHTS & DILEMMAS

_____

_____

_____

_____

_____

_____

_____

_____

_____

_____

The minute you step into the movie theater, it hits you. The popcorn machine. So tempting. I would rationalize that if I bought the giant tub, I could take advantage of their free, second-tub offer. I'd hold the tub in my lap, supposedly sharing it with my family on either side, but of course I wolfed down 80 percent of it. And then being a frugal soul, I got the refill on the way out of the theater and I'd eat the rest at home.

That free tub cost 1,500 calories and 116 grams of fat. Three-thousand calories for a night at the movies!

These days, I bring a handful of almonds, about thirty-five of them. The cost? 170 calories and 15 grams of fat.

DIETER'S DELIGHTS & DILEMMAS

_____

_____

_____

_____

_____

_____

_____

_____

_____

Being outdoors in the crisp, fall weather tends to increase your appetite. We start baking or stocking up on all that Halloween candy in the stores. We fall off the good-health wagon. We eat one, two, three, oh just one more, four, then five cookies. Ummmm, they're so good! Who cares if it's going from lips to hips? From mouth to south.

Maybe you're drowning your pancakes in maple syrup. Remember the cookies and the syrup are mostly sugar. Two small tablespoons of syrup is 460 calories! Okay, so you've done it. (I've done it; I hear your pain.) So stop already. Five cookies?

STOP! The treat is over. Don't keep going. We've fallen, and we **SHALL** get up!

DIETER'S DELIGHTS & DILEMMAS

_____

_____

_____

_____

_____

_____

_____

_____

_____

_____

OCTOBER 10

Chocolate milk has always been my favorite drink. But as I got older, I avoided it because of the high sugar and fat content. But you know what? We can have it! And believe it or not, chocolate milk is an excellent recovery food after a hard workout, say kick boxing, running, weights-then-treadmill . . . any really strenuous workout.

Why? Because we need carbs for energy and protein to help rebuild muscles after such a workout. Cocoa beans also have antioxidants, which also help with muscle repair.

Try skim milk and sugar-free, fat-free, chocolate syrup and enjoy a big, cold glass. Somehow, life is just more fun when you can have chocolate milk.

DIETER'S DELIGHTS & DILEMMAS

_____

_____

_____

_____

_____

_____

_____

_____

_____

I love breakfast. I think it's the variety of the textures, tastes and types of foods that makes breakfast so enjoyable. Did you know that a slice of bacon is better for you than a single sausage link? The calories and fat are almost double in the sausage. One slice of bacon has forty-two calories and three grams of fat, while the sausage has eighty-two calories and seven grams of fat.

A piece of fruit, two eggs, one slice of bacon, a piece of toast and a cup of vanilla tea—what a feast!

But for those die-hard pancake fans, here's a great recipe. Just go easy on the butter or margarine, maple syrup or honey.

HEALTH NUT PANCAKES

3 eggs, separated
1½ cups 2% milk
1¼ cups whole grain wheat flour
¼ cup bran or cornmeal (for texture)
Chopped pecans or walnuts, sesame or sunflower seeds
Canola or sesame oil

Makes 10–12 pancakes

1. *Place the yolks in a large bowl and whip them with a fork. Beat the whites separately in a grease-free bowl until they hold stiff peaks. Stir milk into the yolks, followed by the whole-grain flour and bran or cornmeal. Fold in the beaten egg whites gently with a fork using a light whipping motion until well mixed.*

2. *Oil and heat a griddle. Spoon the batter onto the griddle to form pancakes not more than three inches in diameter so they will cook evenly. Sprinkle top with your choice of nuts or seeds. As the pancakes puff up and begin to bubble on the top, turn them with a flick of the wrist. When the bottoms become dark, they're done.*

OCTOBER 12

L et's call today *choose a treat day*. Every year on my birthday (today) my oldest son Michael gives me a box of Turtles, milk-chocolate-covered pecans and caramel.

My mother loved them and Dad always bought her a box on her birthday as well. I've learned to pace myself. As much as I'd love to eat four or five a day, I only allow myself one Turtle a day.

What is your passion? Dark chocolate pieces? Rice Krispie treats? Try to find something that only has twenty-five to seventy-five calories in each piece and then go ahead—indulge.

If we know we get to satisfy our sweet tooth once a day, it's a good life. Just remember, one. ONE.

DIETER'S DELIGHTS & DILEMMAS

_____

_____

_____

_____

_____

_____

_____

_____

_____

_____

What is success? A six-figure income? A big house, boat, fancy car, huge inheritance? No, success is fulfilling your destiny.

We were all given gifts of talent and free will. Once we discover our talent and create a career using it, the rest is merely doing the work.

We were also given the gift of a lean, strong body. If we've lost it, then we must get it back. We can't be 100 percent at finding success unless we feel good and are strong from within.

Being fat is not fun. It robs us of the ability to think clearly and give 100 percent to living life to the fullest.

We have a goal. We can be successful!

DIETER'S DELIGHTS & DILEMMAS

_____

_____

_____

_____

_____

_____

_____

_____

_____

_____

OCTOBER 14

Studies show that approximately 70 percent of men and 60 percent of women are overweight in America. The weight loss industry is huge.

We spend untold millions of dollars each year trying to lose weight and get fit. We are always looking for that easy way out, that silver lining, that new gadget that will make it easy.

It isn't easy! And if you want the cold, hard truth—the buck stops here. You and me. **We are the only ones who can make us lose weight.** And short of drastic surgery, the only way to do it is to *eat the right foods, eat less food* and *exercise more* than we have in the past.

That's the bottom line.

DIETER'S DELIGHTS & DILEMMAS

_____

_____

_____

_____

_____

_____

_____

_____

_____

W e are a fast-moving nation of people. On the go. Faster, faster. This event, that activity. This class, that meeting. Housework, homework, office work, yard work. We eat standing up, take power naps. We barely have time to brush our teeth, let alone relax for an hour.

If you can't slow down your lifestyle, then at least follow the KISS method of success. Keep It Simple, Sweetie. Make sure you have foods on hand that are fast, easy and always ready for you to pop into your mouth when the hungries hit. You know what they are: Fresh fruit and veggie sticks. Healthy, whole-grain crackers and low-fat cheese. String cheese. Yogurt. Whole-grain breads and peanut butter. **KISS!**

DIETER'S DELIGHTS & DILEMMAS

_____

_____

_____

_____

_____

_____

_____

_____

_____

_____

OCTOBER 16

Who inspires you to maintain a healthy body? My grandfather, William Porter Knapp, who lived well into his nineties, was always a picture of good health. Every morning for breakfast he had a poached egg, a bowl of oatmeal, toast and coffee. He was dead set against drinking and smoking so I'm sure that helped his health as well. In retirement he walked a lot, mostly around his small town in central Illinois, visiting friends and former students. He ate in moderation, all whole foods, many from his large garden out behind the house. The only sweets I remember Grandpa Knapp eating were the lemon drops on the antique buffet in the dining room.

Who inspires you to be healthy?

DIETER'S DELIGHTS & DILEMMAS

_____

_____

_____

_____

_____

_____

_____

_____

_____

_____

Cravings are powerful things. Sometimes I crave popcorn or chocolate, which fall into the snack departments. But other times my body actually craves things like canned beets. I'll eat a whole can, cold, off the shelf. Other times I crave a big, fresh vegetable salad.

If you're craving something that's not good for you, like a large cheese Danish, try to think beyond what that Danish will taste like. How will it make you feel afterward? Full, guilty, stuffed with the wrong kind of fat? If you don't eat it, how will you feel? Proud, powerful, determined? Cravings only last for about twenty minutes. Take a walk, clean the sink, paint your nails, open the mail. Twenty minutes is all.

DIETER'S DELIGHTS & DILEMMAS

Here are two suggestions for our good-eating lifestyle adventure: **Don't ban foods.** You'll only crave them more and more. I gave up candy for Lent and couldn't wait until Easter. I bought a bag of chocolates and ate ten pieces in one hour just after midnight on Easter. Had a hard time sleeping that night.

Forgive and forget. Don't beat yourself up when you eat ten cookies, ten pieces of candy or five pizza slices.

If you say you've gone off your diet, then it feels like you're on a diet. And we aren't! We're on a lifestyle. Let it feel like life.

We'll have our ups and downs but generally it's pretty smooth sailing, right?

DIETER'S DELIGHTS & DILEMMAS

_____

_____

_____

_____

_____

_____

_____

_____

_____

_____

Remember those statistics from October 14 about how many people are overweight in the United States? It's no wonder so many people have diabetes. Type II diabetes means that the body is not producing enough insulin. It's most common if you're over forty and overweight.

Diabetes is just another reason to get serious about this *eating better, eating less, exercising more* weight-loss plan for life. I have friends and relatives who have diabetes. It's so common that probably everyone knows someone with the disease. But who wants to live like that? Worrying every time you eat if it's going to send your blood sugar into the red zone? And those finger pricks? No thank you. Let's eat smart today.

DIETER'S DELIGHTS & DILEMMAS

W e're trying to trim the fat, right? Off our bodies and off those cuts of meat. But remember, we do need a little fat in our diets. It's the teeny, tiny part of the food pyramid, the pointy part at the top.

Fats help transport vitamins A, D, E and K through our bodies. Fats cushion our internal organs. They provide a concentrated source of energy. However, they are very high in calories. One gram of fat equals nine calories, more than double the calories in carbohydrates or protein. We need to eat unsaturated fats only, fats that are liquid at room temperature like sesame, sunflower, olive or Soya oils.

Trim the fat. Blot the bacon. Grill the meat.

DIETER'S DELIGHTS & DILEMMAS

_____

_____

_____

_____

_____

_____

_____

_____

_____

L et's talk about business lunches and dinner meetings. We're not talking social occasions here. We're supposed to be in top form, mentally alert, stunningly creative, full of ideas and bright conversation. So skip the bread, the wine and the dessert.

Eat a small healthy snack just before you go into the lunch or dinner meeting so you won't be tempted to binge on unhealthy appetizers.

Drink water throughout the meeting because alcohol on an empty stomach can give you a headache and make you drowsy or say things you might need to keep to yourself. Avoid dessert so you can be the person with the great ideas at the end of the meal while the others are overindulging.

DIETER'S DELIGHTS & DILEMMAS

_____

_____

_____

_____

_____

_____

_____

_____

_____

_____

I hope you're as proud as I am about the new habits we've developed this year. One of my favorites is drinking a cold bottle of water first thing in the morning when I get up.

It rehydrates me after a long night of sleep and gets my system moving. My other favorite habit is daily exercise. I love getting up and deciding what type of exercise I'll do and what time of day I'll do it.

It's become a routine that's saving my life and my good health. Good habits are so easy to form if you just make up your mind that you'll do something for thirty days. After that the habit is in place.

DIETER'S DELIGHTS & DILEMMAS

_____

_____

_____

_____

_____

_____

_____

_____

_____

Momma always said, "Eat your vegetables." When I was raising my kids I said, "Eat your vegetables." My kids are now saying it to my grandkids.

Vegetables are beautiful, colorful, fun to eat (think corn on the cob!) and very tasty. Vegetables are low in calories, offer lots of dietary fiber, contain valuable nutrients and are known cancer and heart disease protectors. What's not to like about vegetables? Trouble is, we're raising a bunch of kids who want everything to taste like pizza and candy. It's a challenge, but we must teach our children to eat their vegetables if we want our kids to be healthy. Don't give in to the junk food ads. Plant a garden instead.

DIETER'S DELIGHTS & DILEMMAS

_____

_____

_____

_____

_____

_____

Don't you love the idea that we are born with free will? We can make all our own decisions. We're also born with all the tools to have a really great, happy life.

Friends, family, faith, strength of character, health, even the financial means if we work hard. God provides everything we need to grow food: air, sun, soil, wind and rain. We've been given the basics and all the tools. We just have to use these amazing brains we've also been given.

If we cherish these gifts, we can only be winners. We are not junk. We are treasures beyond measure. Let's live up to that today and treat our bodies like rare gems.

DIETER'S DELIGHTS & DILEMMAS

_____

_____

_____

_____

_____

_____

_____

_____

_____

Every few years another diet pill comes on the market. Then a few years later scientists discover that it's dangerous and can lead to greater health problems than being overweight. So they take it off the market. Then something new and improved is invented. Later they find that it has problems.

Give it up! No pill is going to help us get in the lifelong habit of good eating. Why do we want to put chemicals into our magnificent bodies anyway? Who knows what the latest gizmo pill will do to us twenty years from now?

We have the tools to lose weight. We have our brains. We have good, fresh foods. We have determination. Toss the pills!

DIETER'S DELIGHTS & DILEMMAS

_____

_____

_____

_____

_____

_____

_____

_____

_____

_____

OCTOBER 26

Two of the greatest gifts the human race has been given are fresh air and sunshine. On this beautiful fall day, step out of your world. Open the front door and step outside or leave the office for a ten-minute fast walk around the block. Ten minutes of fresh air and sunshine, and you'll be amazed at how it clears your mind and lifts your mood.

Our bodies need it desperately. No wonder people who stay indoors all the time suffer from the depression that accompanies SAD (seasonal affective disorder). Losing weight and getting healthy is all about accepting the gifts that boost our health.

Fresh air and sunshine. Amazing! Are you getting enough?

DIETER'S DELIGHTS & DILEMMAS

_____

_____

_____

_____

_____

Please don't tell my daughter Jeanne, who lives in California and is a natural foods fanatic, that I rarely buy fresh garlic. She lives close to the garlic capitol of the United States and wouldn't think of buying minced garlic in the jar. But I love it.

In fact, I recently purchased a whole quart of minced garlic. I put it in everything . . . soups, stews, salads, pasta dishes, mashed potatoes, meatloaf. Garlic is full of good flavor, plus it's been said that garlic helps prevent flu, colds and viruses. It helps lower cholesterol and is a powerful antibiotic and an antioxidant that protects us from free radicals.

Garlic—another weapon in our arsenal, even the garlic in a jar!

DIETER'S DELIGHTS & DILEMMAS

_____

_____

_____

_____

_____

_____

_____

_____

_____

_____

OCTOBER 28

Here's a good project for all of us. Take a survey. Ask five or ten thin, healthy-looking people of all ages the secret to their *staying thin* lifestyle. Write down their answers.

Many will say, "I only eat when I'm hungry." Or "I eat until I'm full, then I stop." Or "I pay close attention to the types of foods I eat and never overdo it." Or "I work out every day."

But you might get some answers you never thought about before. Write a short article about your survey. Newspapers love survey pieces.

Most importantly, put their answers into your own lifestyle plan. You may find some amazing tricks to staying thin.

DIETER'S DELIGHTS & DILEMMAS

_____

_____

_____

_____

_____

_____

_____

_____

_____

_____

The United Kingdom Tea Council (and who knows more about tea than the Brits?) says tea is so good for us that most people in the UK drink at least four cups a day.

Black or green, tea may reduce the risk of cancer, help control blood pressure, fight viruses and help us live longer. Tea's antioxidants help protect our immune system. If we drink it with skimmed milk it's even healthier because we get a little protein from the milk.

Calm yourself before, during and after a hectic day with a cup of hot tea. I have eighty different flavors on my kitchen shelves, and I keep them in glass jars to protect the flavor.

Tea, anyone?

DIETER'S DELIGHTS & DILEMMAS

October 30

I hate routine. Many people can only function if they have a routine for everything. Those people have it easier when it comes to exercising every day. They schedule it.

My friend Brenda wakes up at six every morning so she can go for an early-morning, wake-up, fast walk or bike ride before the birds start chirping.

Me? I have to remind myself over and over to get on my bike, go for a swim, walk the treadmill, go for a walk.

Whether we schedule our exercise time or do it off the cuff, what's important is that we do it. Off the sofa!

A twenty-minute walk gives us more energy than a twenty-minute nap.

DIETER'S DELIGHTS & DILEMMAS

_____

_____

_____

_____

_____

_____

_____

_____

_____

Trick or treat! Here's a cool trick that's really a treat. You know how an hour before lunch or dinner we get the hungries and we want to chow down on the first thing we can find in the kitchen? Well, try this trick.

Always keep fresh lemons or limes on hand. Squeeze a quarter of a real lemon or lime into a glass of cold water, add a packet of sweetener and ice. Instant fresh lemonade or limeade!

Tall, cool, refreshing and filling enough to hold you to lunch or dinner. A big glass of water or lemonade before dinner is a great way not to overeat.

Remember, we still get a snack after each meal.

DIETER'S DELIGHTS & DILEMMAS

_____

_____

_____

_____

_____

_____

_____

_____

_____

_____

MONTHLY CHECK-IN

Goals Achieved _____

_____

_____

_____

Triggers Pulled and Buttons Pushed_____

_____

_____

_____

Effective Strategies_____

_____

_____

_____

TALE OF THE TAPE

	Current	Last	Net Loss/Gain
Weight	_____	_____	_____
Hips	_____	_____	_____
Thighs	_____	_____	_____
Arms	_____	_____	_____
Waist	_____	_____	_____
Bust	_____	_____	_____

E ver eat a whole package of cookies in one sitting? Or sneak all the mini chocolate candy bars out of your kids' Halloween stash and eat them in one day? Most of us can confess to overeating. Did you know that if you feed goldfish twenty times a day, they'll eat twenty times a day? They'll keep eating until their intestines explode.

If you are fifty or more pounds overweight, you understand the overeating syndrome. It's the most unhealthy thing we can do to our bodies. Talk about sugar overload!

Next time you're tempted to eat the whole bag of candy, tell yourself you can have one piece after each eight-ounce glass of water you drink. Craving gone.

DIETER'S DELIGHTS & DILEMMAS

_____

_____

_____

_____

_____

_____

_____

_____

_____

NOVEMBER 2

Bananas are my new best friend. We can substitute one-quarter cup of mashed bananas for an entire stick of butter and half the sugar in a chocolate-chip cookie recipe and we'll save 1,360 calories per batch!

Speaking of chocolate, remember dark chocolate is much better for us than milk chocolate. There are six times more heart-healthy antioxidants in dark chocolate than in milk chocolate.

Here's more good news . . . light ice cream. They've refined the process and the new light ice creams are delicious, plus they have seven grams less fat and forty milligrams less cholesterol per half cup than regular ice cream.

DIETER'S DELIGHTS & DILEMMAS

_____

_____

_____

_____

_____

_____

_____

_____

_____

L ists make fun reading, as all the popular magazine publishers know. As we fine-tune our year of healthy living through weight reduction and exercise, here's a list of five things *not* to do if we want to live longer. **Don't eat fat, smoke, get stressed, live in pollution or drink alcohol excessively**. And here's a list of thing we *should do* to live longer. **Do move our bodies more often. Do wear seat belts, floss, maintain a PMO (positive mental outlook) and choose our parents well.**

We can control all but the last one of these ten life-extenders. That's the key. We are in control of our lives, our health, our attitudes.

Nobody but us can make us fat, lazy or unhappy.

DIETER'S DELIGHTS & DILEMMAS

_____

_____

_____

_____

_____

_____

_____

_____

_____

_____

Advertising is sneaky. They get us coming and going. For instance, every time I'm at an airport, my nose leads me directly to the Cinnabon place where I inhale deeply, wish desperately I could have one, then, knowing how many hundreds and hundreds of calories and fat they contain, I march past and head for the gate where I'll enjoy the small packet of almonds and raisins I've stashed in my purse. Or, maybe I'll buy a nonfat, fruit yogurt parfait at another fast-food place.

One thing's for sure. Now that I'm so aware of calories taken in and the energy needed to burn them off, I'm not willing to stuff myself with all the not-so-good-for-me foods.

DIETER'S DELIGHTS & DILEMMAS

_____

_____

_____

_____

_____

_____

_____

_____

_____

_____

Get your weekly snacks organized on Sunday night. Buy small plastic food-storage containers and line up ten on the counter and start filling them with healthy snacks to eat throughout the week.

Some may need to be refrigerated. Try nuts, dried fruit, low-fat deli meats, cold cereal, fresh or "light" canned fruit, fat-free yogurt, small chunks of cheese, fresh or canned vegetables. Canned beets sprinkled with a little balsamic vinegar make a delicious snack.

Once you get in the habit of having two snacks and a nutritious lunch each day, you'll be able to avoid the snack machines and you'll start to look and feel marvelous!

DIETER'S DELIGHTS & DILEMMAS

_____

_____

_____

_____

_____

_____

_____

_____

_____

_____

Don't you wish they'd put photos of celebrities on the covers of magazines that were taken the minute they woke up, with no make-up and their hair every which way? Or after a long, hard day when the make-up has run off their faces and all the scars, bags, zits, freckles and age spots make them look like us instead of some impossibly perfect creatures?

I do. At least when someone takes a picture of me I look like a real person with all of the above imperfections. But I always flash my best asset, the one that proclaims to the world just who I am . . . my big toothy smile. It says I am a happy woman—not perfect, just happy.

DIETER'S DELIGHTS & DILEMMAS

_____

_____

_____

_____

_____

_____

_____

_____

_____

This is a yes-and-no world. We have to say **no** to drugs, overspending, fatty and fried foods, second helpings, prejudice, unfair housing . . . the list could go on for days. But we also have to say **yes** to optimism, determination, generosity, love, patience, kindness, learning, persistence, exercise . . . and yes, this list could go on for days.

Losing weight is a yes-and-no proposition as well. We say no to the things that are bad for our bodies and yes to our health and determination to succeed. Losing weight is pretty much a black-and-white, yes-and-no thing. There are few gray areas.

Either you're going to *eat better* foods, *eat less* and *exercise more* or you're not.

DIETER'S DELIGHTS & DILEMMAS

H ow many times do you eat out each week, counting restaurant meals, fast-food meals and lunches grabbed out of vending machines?

Most Americans eat out an average of five times a week. I average only two to three times out of twenty-one meals a week.

The average restaurant meal contains at least 1,000 calories. If we're trying to keep our calories to 1,500 or 1,800 a day, that's a big part of our daily intake and doesn't leave much room for the other two major meals and three snacks a day. The solutions?

Choose foods wisely in restaurants. Bring at least half of the meal home and have it the next day for lunch. Avoid buffets and high-fat items at salad bars.

DIETER'S DELIGHTS & DILEMMAS

_____

_____

_____

_____

_____

_____

_____

_____

_____

British Prime Minister William Gladstone wrote, *If you're cold, tea will warm you. If you're heated, it will cool you. If you're depressed, it will cheer you. If you're excited, it will calm you.*

As an inveterate tea drinker, I know it's all true. I also think Gladstone's words apply to a good brisk walk. If you're cold, a fast walk will certainly warm you up. If you're hot, the fresh air, especially this time of year, will cool you off. If you're depressed, walking raises endorphins and you'll feel better emotionally. If you're angry, excited, or stressed, a fast walk will calm you down.

Try it. In fact, try it every day.

DIETER'S DELIGHTS & DILEMMAS

_____

_____

_____

_____

_____

_____

_____

_____

_____

_____

Time for self-introspection. Ask yourself, *What am I? An overeater? An underexerciser? An oversnacker? Under-water-drinker? Overplanner? Undermotivator?*

We need to know what our strengths and weaknesses are when it comes to losing weight effectively. I know I'm an overeater after dinner at night. I'm also an underexerciser. My two weak areas. After dinner in front of the TV, I can find more excuses to eat, eat, eat. I know that, and now I'm trying very hard to change that bad habit.

Now, I often take a walk around the block when the cravings hit. Or I work on crafts that keep my hands busy.

DIETER'S DELIGHTS & DILEMMAS

_____

_____

_____

_____

_____

_____

_____

_____

How many magazine articles are we going to read about dieting? Every month, health, fitness and women's magazines have to find more and more articles on the subject because we are obsessed with it.

First it was "don't eat breads and starches." Then we were told, "Don't eat fat." Next came, "Don't eat carbs," and "Eat mostly meat and fat." We can't fall for it. It's how publishers sell magazines. Hope for a new weight-loss secret is a powerful tease, but the only thing that works to take weight off is eating less than our body needs to maintain our weight.

To lose fat, not muscle, we need to lose slowly, no more than a pound or two a week. It's that simple.

DIETER'S DELIGHTS & DILEMMAS

_____

_____

_____

_____

_____

_____

_____

_____

_____

How many calories a day do we need to maintain our weight? Simply multiply your weight by ten.

If you weigh 240 pounds, you need 2,400 calories a day to maintain that weight. Eat more, you'll gain weight. Eat less, you'll lose weight.

One pound equals 3,500 calories. If you eliminate 500 calories a day you'll lose about a pound every seven days.

If you weigh 150, you only need 1,500 calories per day to maintain that weight. If you reduce that by 250 calories a day, you'll lose about a pound every fourteen days, or two pounds a month.

DIETER'S DELIGHTS & DILEMMAS

November is so often a cold, gray month, at least in many places in our country. Today, I want to give you a special treat . . . the easiest cake to make and one of the most delicious. Pineapple shortcake.

Simply mix one angel-food cake mix and one twenty-ounce can of crushed pineapple. Pour into a large sheet-cake pan and bake for thirty minutes at 350 degrees until the top is golden brown. Put any kind of fruit on top just before you serve it and top with two tablespoons of nonfat, dairy topping.

Remember, eat just one small piece of cake, and a half cup of fruit. It's all about portion control, remember? Enjoy this bit of sunshine!

DIETER'S DELIGHTS & DILEMMAS

NOVEMBER 14

If you're just starting your weight-loss plan this week, welcome to the world of better health. Remember, it's much better to lose pounds slowly because it's the fat that goes, not the muscle.

But if you want to jump-start it for a few days, try substituting lunch or dinner with a bowl of wholesome cereal and skim milk. Don't do this for more than a week because your body will tire of the routine and start craving more fruits and vegetables, protein and other carbohydrates.

Isn't it amazing that our bodies actually let us know when they need a certain vitamin or mineral by making us crave it?

DIETER'S DELIGHTS & DILEMMAS

_____

_____

_____

_____

_____

_____

_____

_____

_____

_____

Before the big Turkey Day feast, let's try to get in the habit of choosing the right proportions of food. Visualize a dinner plate. Divide it in half. Fill one half with fresh, cooked vegetables. No sauces, just good wholesome vegetables, perhaps two different kinds. Broccoli and carrots. Or cauliflower and green beans.

Divide the other half of the plate into two halves or two one-quarter sections. In one of those, place your meat or protein food. In the other half, your carbs or starch food. A fresh, dark-green salad can go on its own separate bowl or small plate.

Remember our goals. Eat less, eat slowly, talk more, enjoy your company. Eating is a social event.

DIETER'S DELIGHTS & DILEMMAS

_____

_____

_____

_____

_____

_____

_____

_____

_____

_____

November 16

Whether you're baking pies for Thanksgiving or just planning to eat them, here are some pie facts. A slice of pumpkin pie (one-eighth of a nine-inch pie) has 220 calories, 26 carbs and 11 grams of fat. My favorite, pecan, has a whopping 610 calories for the same size slice, 62 carbs and 39 grams of fat. Excess butter is the culprit here.

But if you're like me and can't live without one slice of Grandma Bev's amazing pecan pie, go ahead. Just be thankful you can say no to a second helping and go for a nice, long walk in the crisp fall air.

Enjoy the holidays. Just make good choices.

DIETER'S DELIGHTS & DILEMMAS

I've watched them in restaurants. Overweight people are generally fast eaters. They dive in, shovel away, rarely put the fork down and talk very little during the meal. Thin people tend to eat slower and are more social. I'm somewhere in between, but I'm going to slow it down even more.

Why eat slowly? It's a no-brainer. Your brain tells you you're full long before you eat *the whole thing* and hopefully you'll stop eating when full. Having a hard time slowing down? If you're right-handed, eat with your left hand for a week. Or the opposite if you're left-handed. Or try eating with chopsticks for a week.

Today, and always, **slow down!** You'll eat less and enjoy it more.

DIETER'S DELIGHTS & DILEMMAS

_____

_____

_____

_____

_____

_____

_____

_____

_____

Are you a late-night snacker like I am? I do fine around 8 or 9 P.M. with a small 100-calorie snack, perhaps yogurt, sugar-free pudding, or celery and peanut butter.

But then if I'm still up at 11 P.M. or midnight and I get one tiny little hunger pang, I'm off to the kitchen for chips, candy or last night's left-over dessert. I know it reverses all the good, healthy eating I've done all day.

So how do I stop? One cup of herbal tea. Or one-half piece of toast with one teaspoon of peanut butter. Or one-half granola bar.

Best idea: a glass of ice water that will fill me up long enough to get my well-fed body to bed.

DIETER'S DELIGHTS & DILEMMAS

I t isn't enough to do aerobic exercise. We all need a little weight training to go along with it if we want strong, long, lean, effective muscles.

Try keeping a set of five- to ten-pound dumbbells next to your TV chair. Tell yourself that you'll do arm presses, forward and backward, during all the commercials.

Or strap a five-pound lead weight to your remote control. Lead is very dense and weighs a lot per square inch. Tape a lead weight to your hairbrush, your cell phone, anything you use a lot during the day.

Each time we lift something with weights added to it, we become stronger and more heart healthy.

DIETER'S DELIGHTS & DILEMMAS

NOVEMBER 20

This year for Thanksgiving, let's make a deal. No taste-testing in the kitchen before dinner. Eat slowly. Enjoy the conversation during the big meal with our loved ones. No second helpings. Help with the dishes. Then invite the whole gang, the ones not glued to the football games on TV, to go for a walk. A long walk. Talk, sing, solve the family's problems.

Or, if you're really ambitious, start a family tradition after dinner of a touch football game, a game of softball or go sledding if you live in snow country.

Get your friends and family into the active habit. Talk about it at dinner tonight.

Let's make this Thanksgiving the year we begin some healthy traditions.

DIETER'S DELIGHTS & DILEMMAS

_____
_____
_____
_____
_____
_____
_____
_____
_____
_____

One study says spicy foods may help boost our metabolism, which helps burn more calories. I'm basically a healthy person with a healthy digestion, strong bones and good blood pressure. I do need to lose more weight and get my cholesterol down, but I think my love of spicy foods helps keep my metabolism in good shape. I love to cook with cayenne pepper, curry, hot sauce, horseradish, salsa, hot peppers, all sorts of spicy foods.

Start with a teaspoon of green Tabasco sauce in soups, salad dressings and pasta dishes. It's so mild no one will ever know, but it adds flavor and boosts your metabolism. And here's an easy recipe for horseradish—horseradish root is in the produce section.

FRESH HORSERADISH

1 root of fresh horseradish
½ cup white vinegar
2 teaspoons salt

*Makes
2 cups*

1. *Using a vegetable peeler, scrape any discolored spots from a root of fresh horseradish. Cut it into cubes approximately 1 inch in size. Finely chop the cubes using a blender or food processor. Mix with the white vinegar and salt.*
2. *Pack into clean, well-scrubbed jars, cover tightly and allow to ripen in the refrigerator for a week before serving. Once the container is opened, the horseradish loses its strength quickly.*

A re you a coffee-holic? Many people, especially those in large cities, depend on expensive brews to get them through the day. Problem is, they keep ordering more and more luxurious brews with more cream and sugar than coffee.

Many are over 500 calories each, not counting the whipped cream on top. Give up one 500-calorie extra-rich, high-fat, high-sugared latte a day and you could lose fifty pounds a year.

As the days get shorter and the weather gets colder, a tall mocha warms our hands and soothes our cravings. But don't get in the habit. Try a large cup of Chai tea, some honey and skim milk. Less caffeine, so you'll sleep better too.

DIETER'S DELIGHTS & DILEMMAS

_____

_____

_____

_____

_____

_____

_____

_____

_____

Ever notice how if we write it down, we tend to do it? The most helpful and healthful writing I do is when I write on my calendar how many lengths of the pool I swim each day.

I started out with ten, then twenty. *I can do more,* I said to myself. The next day I did thirty. I wrote it down. When I looked at the calendar I was inspired to keep improving.

The next day I did forty. By the end of the following week, I'd been swimming for an hour and did eighty lengths, which I proudly wrote on my calendar in red ink.

Get a calendar and write down your accomplishments.

DIETER'S DELIGHTS & DILEMMAS

_____

_____

_____

_____

_____

_____

_____

_____

_____

NOVEMBER 24

Eating sensibly is hard when we're trying to cut back our portion sizes. At breakfast, especially, two poached eggs on a plate look smaller than two peas on a platter if you're really hungry. So plump up the volume! Plump up the fiber!

Scramble those eggs with a quarter cup of skim milk, then add spinach, onions, garlic, mushrooms, tomatoes . . . any combo of fresh veggies. You won't add many calories because we all know fresh vegetables are very low in the calorie department, and the milk adds a little bit of "good-for-you" fat, calcium and some protein. In addition to a much bigger volume of food, you'll be getting lots of good fiber.

Plump it up!

DIETER'S DELIGHTS & DILEMMAS

We need thirty grams of fiber a day. Sometimes it's hard, especially if we're not eating as many fresh vegetables and fresh fruits as we should. I make sure I get most of my fiber in the morning when I eat my homemade granola.

I have a huge stainless-steel bowl where I mix all the following ingredients. Three pounds of granola from the health food store and then two cups each of oat bran, wheat bran, walnuts, wheat germ, sunflower seeds, raisins, craisins and a box of Bran Buds. Mix it well and store in airtight containers.

I'm probably getting enough fiber in a bowl of my doctored-up granola to build a boat!

DIETER'S DELIGHTS & DILEMMAS

_____

_____

_____

_____

_____

_____

_____

_____

_____

_____

Sometimes it seems our nation is obsessed with booze. Alcohol contains empty calories and can therefore put on the pounds. It can damage vital organs. Plus, it's expensive.

Next time you're in a social situation where everyone is consuming alcoholic drinks, try something different. Ask for a club soda with lemon or a diet cola with a splash of vanilla extract. Or squeeze a quarter of a whole lime into a tall glass of ice tea.

Often we drink those mixed, alcoholic drinks simply because they taste so good. Chocolate martinis and orange-blossom specials taste just as good without the alcohol, and if you ask for sugar-free drinks, they have fewer calories and, best of all, no hangover.

DIETER'S DELIGHTS & DILEMMAS

Why let the stress of the holidays, the parties, presents, pandemonium and pressure turn us into crazed zombies who can never do enough to make the season bright?

Let's enjoy every day. Whether we're celebrating Christmas, Hanukkah, Kwanzaa, Chinese New Year, or any other holiday on the calendar this time of year, let's try to make these days simpler. We aren't going to fall for the "I have to buy the best presents and spend the most money to impress my friends and family" temptations. Take a deep breath, call a family meeting and discuss the holiday season. Expectations. Plans. Traditions. Divide the work. Double the pleasure. Our mental and physical health is important.

DIETER'S DELIGHTS & DILEMMAS

_____

_____

_____

_____

_____

_____

_____

_____

_____

L ook in the mirror. Do you look better physically than you did a year ago? Do you feel better inside?

If you've lost weight, chances are people are noticing the new you. Do you get compliments left and right? Feels good, doesn't it?

Today, let's step out of ourselves and find *someone else* to compliment. I often see someone in a crowd who is inspiring . . . an older man with a wonderful smile, a harried, young mother who treats her children with respect in a difficult situation in a department store, a woman with beautiful, healthy skin and hair.

Remember, one compliment from a stranger can make the entire day a good one. Pass it on!

DIETER'S DELIGHTS & DILEMMAS

_____

_____

_____

_____

_____

_____

_____

_____

_____

I've worked hard all year, but my midriff and stomach still stick out way too far. I have to admit I perk up when I hear or see something about a magic bullet that can do the work for me. Chewing gum that's supposed to help me lose weight. No-calorie mints that trick my mouth. Flavor sprays that supposedly replace all the heavy sauces in my life. Extra-thick, "weight-loss" lip gloss that's so gooey I don't want to put food anywhere near my lips! Even aroma patches that distract me from tempting food smells.

Gimmicks, every one. Face it. We just have to tough it out. *Eat better*, more nutritious foods, *eat less* and *exercise more.* It's simple. It works.

DIETER'S DELIGHTS & DILEMMAS

_____

_____

_____

_____

_____

_____

_____

_____

_____

_____

It's turkey salad time. If you cooked Thanksgiving dinner this year, you probably have enough leftover turkey to feed half the fire department.

Cut the turkey in bite-size pieces and add lots of healthy vegetables and spices. Celery, onions, green pepper, garlic, a dash or two of hot sauce, sweet-hot peppers chopped up and a quarter-cup of fat-free ranch dressing to give it a creamy texture. Eat it on whole-grain bread laced with a dark green leaf lettuce.

The protein and fiber from this lunch will keep us feeling full for hours. No fair munching on the leftover Turkey Day pies, cakes or candies. If you need something sweet, eat a half cup of fat-free yogurt with a half cup of fresh fruit.

DIETER'S DELIGHTS & DILEMMAS

_____

_____

_____

_____

_____

_____

_____

_____

_____

Nothing tastes better on a cold winter morning than a big bowl of hot oatmeal. We've all seen the commercials about how oatmeal can help lower our cholesterol levels. It's true. And there's a lot more to oatmeal than that.

Oatmeal contains manganese, which is essential for the utilization of vitamin B. It's got omega 3 fatty acids, tryptophan (an essential amino acid), vitamin K (which helps with bone loss and controls blood clotting) and phosphorus (an essential element that forms the backbone for our DNA). Oatmeal is loaded with dietary fiber. Overall, it's an amazing food.

Eat up! It's cold out there.

DIETER'S DELIGHTS & DILEMMAS

_____

_____

_____

_____

_____

_____

_____

_____

_____

_____

DECEMBER 2

We know all about those goofy magazine ads that promise you can lose ten pounds in one week. We know that what you lose is mostly water and muscle tissue (and temporarily, at that), but very little fat.

Any high-protein diet high in fat, saturated fat and cholesterol (which is the standard of the low-carb diets) is a dangerous thing. It's like they're cutting down the forest to save a tree.

Over-the-top protein diets can easily lead to heart disease, kidney and colon problems, and pack on the cholesterol in our bloodstream. Wow. Sometimes we just have to be smarter than that.

DIETER'S DELIGHTS & DILEMMAS

_____

_____

_____

_____

_____

_____

_____

_____

_____

_____

Years ago, I saw an article about the top twelve most perfect foods—the dynamite dozen I like to call them.

Amazingly, none of these twelve perfect foods are on the list when you ask kids to write down their favorite foods. Kids want burgers, fries, chicken nuggets, macaroni and cheese, shakes, soda, chips, pizza, candy, cakes, brownies and ice cream. The perfect foods? Whole-grain breads, skim milk, nuts, fish, beans, prunes, bananas, peppers, carrots, brown rice, tofu and tomatoes.

If we could give up the first list and eat heartily from the second list, we'd sure be fit and fabulous when it comes to good health, wouldn't we?

DIETER'S DELIGHTS & DILEMMAS

DECEMBER 4

During the winter months we tend to eat heavier foods. Bigger breakfasts may include bacon or ham and eggs cooked in the bacon grease. Pizza sounds good on a cold December night. Even burgers might be cooking on the stove.

Get out the paper towels and start blotting. As soon as the cooking is finished, start blotting. Blot all the extra fat and grease off the food you're going to eat. You'll be surprised how much fat you can blot up. It's better for that fat to land in a paper towel than inside your arteries clogging things up.

Better yet, grill that meat. Or cook bacon in the microwave between paper towels. You'll see how much grease there is.

DIETER'S DELIGHTS & DILEMMAS

We've talked about how it takes the body twelve to twenty minutes to tell us we're full after we start eating. So a half-hour before dinner when you're ravenous and ready to eat Milwaukee, give yourself a nutritious snack that will curb your appetite.

Drink six ounces of V-8 juice. Or whip up a small fruit smoothie in the blender. Eight ounces of plain yogurt, a tablespoon of honey, a piece of fresh fruit and a few ice cubes and you've got a nutritious, low-cal snack that will most definitely keep you from overeating during dinner.

I love the idea that I'm finally figuring my body out, and overeating is not what it wants.

DIETER'S DELIGHTS & DILEMMAS

_____

_____

_____

_____

_____

_____

_____

_____

_____

_____

DECEMBER 6

As temperatures drop, my need for hot drinks and chocolate increases. When I'm traveling, especially, I often long for a nice cup of hot chocolate to warm me up. So I buy those individual servings of instant hot chocolate, the no-sugar, no-fat kind and keep them in my purse, travel bag and backpack. Carry a couple plastic spoons with you and ask for a cup of hot water at the airport or on a plane, at the office or train station.

It's all about preplanning. And if we make our cocoa with skim milk, we're getting a protein bonus as well. See how much fun it is to lose weight and get warm at the same time?

DIETER'S DELIGHTS & DILEMMAS

_____

_____

_____

_____

_____

_____

_____

_____

_____

L et's make today Big Pot Day. Get out the biggest pot you own or borrow one. Make up a huge batch of something nutritious and delicious like vegetable soup with twenty different vegetables. Think how much fun you'll have in the produce department buying them all. Or make chicken-noodle soup with celery, onions, carrots, garlic and parsley.

After you've cooked the big pot of soup or chili, divide it into individual serving sizes and freeze them. Then, when you need a quick meal, pop the container into the microwave.

My big pot holds ten quarts. Cooking healthy meals ten quarts at a time is more fun than one quart a day.

DIETER'S DELIGHTS & DILEMMAS

_____

_____

_____

_____

_____

_____

_____

_____

_____

_____

DECEMBER 8

Every so often we need one or two days to jump-start our weight-loss program back into high gear. Cutting four to five hundred calories out of our eating for a couple days may kick our metabolism back into running at peak level.

If you're a medium-sized woman, eating 1,800 calories a day to lose weight at a nice, safe, slow pace, you might want to cut back to 1,400. On those days think *three + one = four + one = five*. Three hundred for breakfast, 100 for a snack, 400 for lunch, 100 for a snack and 500 for dinner.

It's still plenty of calories for good nutrition, but at just 1,400 total, you'll lose weight, especially if you're also exercising for thirty to forty-five minutes a day.

DIETER'S DELIGHTS & DILEMMAS

_____

_____

_____

_____

_____

_____

_____

_____

_____

Seems like I eat more fat in the winter. Perhaps I'm confused with hibernating bears and whale blubber. Now is a good time to concentrate on eating only good-for-us fats.

In one study, 20 percent of the calories eaten were from the good monounsaturated fats like nuts, peanut butter, olive oil and avocados. Another group received 35 percent of their calories from these good fats.

The people in both groups lost an average of eleven pounds that first year, but the group that got 35 percent of their calories from the good fats were able to keep the weight off for eighteen months or longer.

So the good fats are important.

DIETER'S DELIGHTS & DILEMMAS

_____

_____

_____

_____

_____

_____

_____

_____

_____

L ow-carb diets are losing ground because they tend to make people compulsive eaters who wouldn't touch an apple if it was an archery target on top of their head.

When you eat too much protein you're actually depleting muscle fluids. In reality 50–60 percent of your daily calories should come from the good carbohydrates: whole grains, fruits and vegetables, but none or very few from the bad carbs: anything made from white sugar, white flour, or white shortening.

Again, it's that nasty word, "diet" that steers us in the wrong direction. We don't ever want to go on a diet. We're on a good-nutrition, good-exercise plan for life, remember?

DIETER'S DELIGHTS & DILEMMAS

_____

_____

_____

_____

_____

_____

_____

_____

_____

_____

The holiday season with all its expectations often opens a giant can of depression. Here are four ideas to help make it better.

1. Start a new tradition. Do things differently than in past holidays.

2. Do something for someone else, a stranger. Giving time to others is truly the way to beat depression.

3. Stop self-induced physical abuse. If you're eating too much sugar, fat and alcohol, get out there every morning and fast walk. A moment on the lips, a lifetime on the hips is not worth it.

4. Be more childlike. Make a mess when you bake cookies. Lie in the snow and make snow angels. Organize a gift exchange. Go caroling.

DIETER'S DELIGHTS & DILEMMAS

_____

_____

_____

_____

_____

_____

_____

_____

_____

_____

DECEMBER 12

It's tough watching those trays of high-cal, high-fat foods float by at holiday parties, but we can celebrate and enjoy the festivities and still stay healthy:

Eat this: Two tablespoons of salsa (9 calories, 0 grams of fat). *Not this*: two tablespoons of guacamole (55 calories, 5 grams of fat).

Eat this: Twelve large shrimp with one-quarter cup of cocktail sauce (165 calories, less than 1 gram of fat). *Not this:* one crab cake (290 calories, 19 grams of fat).

Eat this: Three chocolate Hershey Kisses (75 calories, 8 carbs). *Not this:* A half-cup of M&Ms (256 calories, 37 carbs).

It's all about choices.

DIETER'S DELIGHTS & DILEMMAS

_____

_____

_____

_____

_____

_____

_____

_____

_____

_____

I know some families who have pizza at least one night a week. It's a fitness buster waiting to happen because usually the white, nutritionless crust is topped with greasy meats and enough fatty cheese to run strings around town and back.

Make your own pizza, packed with power and nutrition. These days you can buy 100 percent whole-grain, thin crusts, ready-made. Top with a thin layer of fat-free mozzarella cheese, then go to town with the fresh veggies and low-fat meats. My favorite includes shrimp, Thai peanut sauce, bean sprouts, stringed carrots, green onion tops and dry-roasted peanuts. It's an Asian delight pizza, packed with low-fat, low-carb protein. Good enough for company.

DIETER'S DELIGHTS & DILEMMAS

DECEMBER 14

Did you ever play that game, "which would you rather be, beautiful or smart? Creative or perfectly proportioned? Rich or thin? Talented or healthy?"

Well, we can have it all. We've learned all year how to be thinner and healthy. To be beautiful we just have to flash our best smile and treat others with kindness. Beauty comes from within. We can develop talents because we're all born with many talents. And we can use our newfound healthy energy to work harder on the job and we'll be rich in many ways, not just financially.

It's all up to us. We have the keys. We can do it. Stay with the program.

DIETER'S DELIGHTS & DILEMMAS

F eeling stressed? Rushed? "To-do" list too long and overwhelming? Time for a little at-home spa action.

Mix a bit of oatmeal with brown sugar and gently rub it over your face for a natural exfoliating scrub. Soak your feet in sudsy warm water, then use a pumice stone to soften the calluses. Save your next two tea bags and put them in the refrigerator in a sealed plastic bag so they stay damp. When chilled, place them on your eyelids to reduce puffiness while you relax in the recliner. A nice, long, hot bath should finish up your day or evening at the home spa.

Isn't it great how many inexpensive, fun ways there are to pamper yourself?

DIETER'S DELIGHTS & DILEMMAS

DECEMBER 16

No matter what your faith background is, this seems to be the time of year when people celebrate with parties, decorations, gifts, religious customs and fancy dinners. It's a good thing. We need something to perk up these short days and long, cold nights. We need all the celebration we can get. We just don't need the excessive calories, fats, sugar and alcohol consumption.

We need to hold on to our senses and stay healthy. If you find yourself reaching for one more holiday cookie or one more gooey appetizer, think! Start up an interesting conversation instead. We're surrounded with people, new friends and old friends this time of year. Get acquainted. Talk, don't eat.

DIETER'S DELIGHTS & DILEMMAS

Did you ever meet someone whose idea of weight loss is to eat just one big meal a day? I can't imagine how anyone could go all day without eating and then stuff themselves at a big dinner in the evening.

I asked my doctor about it and he said that starving, then eating a large meal makes the body release high levels of insulin. And that's not good for the body. In fact, it can be downright dangerous. Our bodies need food to function. They need a nice steady stream of good-for-you food while we're awake and working or playing.

During the holiday season, especially, we need to treat our bodies well. No junk. Good healthy eating.

DIETER'S DELIGHTS & DILEMMAS

_____

_____

_____

_____

_____

_____

_____

_____

_____

_____

DECEMBER 18

If you're like me, you have to think about not over-eating every single day. Unlike my naturally thin friends, I think about food often, probably every hour I'm awake. Maybe it's because I work at home and can walk to the kitchen on a second's notice and start rambling through the cupboards and refrigerator.

When did I eat last? Was it a snack or a meal? Should I eat half the leftovers or all of them for lunch? Do I feel like making a salad? Why shouldn't I have a cup full of Chex Mix? Often I satisfy my food thoughts by making myself a cup of tea or ice tea.

It's always a struggle. But we can do it.

DIETER'S DELIGHTS & DILEMMAS

_____

_____

_____

_____

_____

_____

_____

_____

_____

America seems obsessed with its overweight problem, especially with the morbidly obese. They parade them out during the major TV talk shows and talk about how their condition causes depression, joint pain, type II diabetes, hypertension, shortness of breath and sleep apnea.

The audience wants to know how these people can let themselves get that fat. We, who have been over-eaters most of our lives, can understand how. Pack-a-day smokers who can't stop understand how. Drug users who can't shake the habit understand how. It takes time, counseling and gut-wrenching determination and steel will. We have it. Every single day is one step forward.

DIETER'S DELIGHTS & DILEMMAS

_____

_____

_____

_____

_____

_____

_____

_____

_____

L osing lots of weight in a short time so we can fit into that wedding gown or impress the folks at our class reunion or look great in a swimsuit doesn't work.

Why be so miserable starving yourself when you're only going to gain all that weight back and then some in a few months? Dr. Phil said our chance of dying from a heart attack is 70 percent greater for those on yo-yo diets. Lose a lot, gain it back. Lose it again, gain even more back. At the end of the year you're worse off than when you started.

We must do it slowly. Slowly, but consistently.

DIETER'S DELIGHTS & DILEMMAS

_____

_____

_____

_____

_____

_____

_____

_____

_____

Our bodies are strange and wonderful things. Stress can make us hold onto weight. So can feelings of hurt or anger. Depression can practically shut down the body's ability to shed pounds, often because when we're depressed we don't have the energy to work out or even go for a walk around the block.

The body senses something's wrong and holds onto the extra weight for self-preservation. When all systems are working smoothly, there's no serious physical or mental illness and we're getting plenty of daily exercise, our bodies are free to let go and break down those fat cells and flush them out of the body.

Get healthy mentally and your body will follow.

DIETER'S DELIGHTS & DILEMMAS

DECEMBER 22

Here's a holiday gift for you. The world's five healthiest foods according to *Health Magazine*.

1. **Olive oil.** It helps control LDL, the bad cholesterol and raises HDL, the good cholesterol.
2. **Soy (tofu).** The Japanese eat 60–120 grams a day while Americans eat practically zero.
3. **Yogurt.** It promotes intestinal health, builds strong bones and may even help with weight loss.
4. **Lentils.** Think protein, iron, fiber, antioxidants and loads of vitamins.
5. **Kimchi.** This fermented cabbage, loaded with vitamins and healthy bacteria, keeps obesity at bay in Korea where they eat it in practically everything.

DIETER'S DELIGHTS & DILEMMAS

_____

_____

_____

_____

_____

_____

_____

_____

_____

I saw a television show where a woman was considering having plastic surgery to reduce the size of her calves. She said her husband didn't think they were sexy enough and he couldn't even look at her in the shower.

The woman, who was wearing slacks, was a tall, thin, drop-dead gorgeous, smart blond who seemed devastated by her husband's feelings about her legs. The host scolded her, "If you're trying to lose weight for your husband or your parents or your friends, anyone who seems judgmental of you, stop it right there!"

We can only lose weight for ourselves, because we want to be healthier, because we want to feel good.

Make sure you're doing it for *you*.

DIETER'S DELIGHTS & DILEMMAS

_____

_____

_____

_____

_____

_____

_____

_____

_____

DECEMBER 24

During this year we've worked on all the areas of our life . . . *Social, Physical, Emotional, Career, Intellectual, Environmental* and *Spiritual*. We are whole beings, interesting, changeable, constantly learning. The flesh that hangs on our bones is just the packaging. There's a whole amazing being underneath.

Yes, we want our packages to look as beautiful as the most gorgeous boxes under the tree. But remember, it's what's inside that counts. Let's try not to get so caught up in resculpting ourselves that we forget the other important elements of our life.

Our essence or spirit is the only thing that lasts for eternity. Be happy. Love others as you want to be loved and watch it come back to you.

DIETER'S DELIGHTS & DILEMMAS

Take away the commercialization of Christmas and what do we have? Hope. Joy. Giving. Families and friends together. Games. Laughter. It isn't about putting on the dog for influential people. It isn't about how many cookies we bake or how many gifts we wrap. It's much simpler than that. It's about loving ourselves enough to avoid the stressful, overeating parts of the holiday season and wanting to spend more time with people we enjoy, love, and care about.

This is the season when we truly step outside ourselves and give quality time to others. It's the season where we get to think about the past year and make plans for the next one. Be merry this Christmas day.

DIETER'S DELIGHTS & DILEMMAS

_____

_____

_____

_____

_____

_____

_____

_____

_____

DECEMBER 26

If you had too many helpings of holiday cheer yesterday, don't beat yourself up today. Dust yourself off, step on that scale, and for the next week write down an estimate of all the calories you consume.

By the end of the year you'll have an idea of how much food you're really consuming, then, come January 1, you can step on that scale, write down the amount of weight you need to lose and get busy. The beauty of being a healthful eater is that little failures here and there are not permanent.

A new way of eating and looking at food is: We're on our way to feeling better every day!

DIETER'S DELIGHTS & DILEMMAS

_____

_____

_____

_____

_____

_____

_____

_____

_____

Both our brains and our bodies atrophy with lack of use. If we sit around watching TV and rarely exercise, our muscles get smaller, our bodies shrink, and we become weak.

It's what happens to many people in their eighties and nineties. They stop exercising. Often, they stop reading, studying, trying to solve problems or learn new skills. Eventually, they lose interest in most things around them and become unable to have interesting conversations. We don't have to let it happen.

Our bodies and our brains need exercise every day. Give your favorite oldster a puzzle book. Take him for a walk. And remember, when we get old, we'll exercise both body and brain, right?

DIETER'S DELIGHTS & DILEMMAS

DECEMBER 28

Women, especially, seem to pay close attention to all those ads and products that advertise alpha-hydroxy acids, the magical ingredients that are supposed to reduce tiny facial lines and fade age spots. Here's the big secret. AHA is made from the juices of citric acid fruits like oranges and grapefruit.

AHA can help reverse sun damage to skin and give us a more youthful glow to our skin, but why don't we just drink the real thing . . . more orange and grapefruit juice to get the same benefits? AHA cannot get rid of deep lines or sags. Quitting smoking, regular exercise and losing weight will help with those.

Today, let's try some fresh-squeezed orange juice for breakfast.

DIETER'S DELIGHTS & DILEMMAS

We're smack dab in the middle of the holidays. Perhaps we've fallen off the wagon of good eating habits. Stand in front of a full-length mirror. Body image is about what we see and what we think about what we see. It's about our feelings about how we look and about whether or not our bodies function well. Does your back ache, or your knees or hips hurt when you walk? How do others react to our bodies?

We are the only ones who can change our body image. We can change it! We can eat the right foods today, in smaller portions. We can get outside and move that body. Yes, we can!

DIETER'S DELIGHTS & DILEMMAS

December 30

How are you doing? If you've been working on a healthy-eating program since last January you should see real results, not only on the scale, but in your energy level, your general health, your attitude about when and how much to eat, and about the importance of daily exercise.

In the space below, write down the changes in YOU since last January. Remember, the beauty of all this is if you've lost weight slowly this year, it's because you have adopted a whole new, healthy lifestyle. Slow is best and if you've just begun your "new you" lifestyle, a whole new year starts day after tomorrow!

This plan never ends. It's ongoing, year after year.

Here's to your good health!

DIETER'S DELIGHTS & DILEMMAS

_____

_____

_____

_____

_____

_____

_____

_____

_____

We did it! An entire year of motivation, celebration, inspiration. If you've fallen off the stage, jump right back on. Remember, this is an eating plan for life.

Protecting our good health is the single most important thing we can do with our lives. We've learned to eat better foods, eat fewer foods and move our bodies as they were intended to move. Our battle cry is *eat better, eat less, exercise more.* If we follow this for life, we will be healthy.

Happy New Year! Let's start again tomorrow and every New Year's day. We can do it. We can lose weight, stand tall and be proud of ourselves and the glorious bodies we've nurtured. *Bravo!*

DIETER'S DELIGHTS & DILEMMAS

_____

_____

_____

_____

_____

_____

_____

_____

_____

MONTHLY CHECK-IN

Goals Achieved _____

_____

_____

_____

Triggers Pulled and Buttons Pushed _____

_____

_____

_____

Effective Strategies _____

_____

_____

_____

TALE OF THE TAPE

	Current	Last	Net Loss/Gain
Weight	_____	_____	_____
Hips	_____	_____	_____
Thighs	_____	_____	_____
Arms	_____	_____	_____
Waist	_____	_____	_____
Bust	_____	_____	_____